ConsumerReports®

The Best *of* Health

270 Questions you've always wanted to ask your doctor

Marvin M. Lipman, M.D.,
and the Editors of
Consumer Reports on Health

Consumer Reports Best of Health is published by Consumer Reports, the nonprofit organization that publishes *Consumer Reports*, the monthly magazine of test reports, product Ratings, and buying guidance. Established in 1936, Consumer Reports chartered under the Not-for-Profit Corporation Law of the State of New York. Standard postage paid at White Plains, NY, and at other mailing offices. Canadian postage paid at Mississauga, Ontario, Canada. Canadian publications registration no. 2665247-98; agreement number PM40015148. U.S. Postmaster: Send address changes to P.O. Box 2109, Harlan, IA 51593-0298. Canada Post: If copies are undeliverable, return to Consumer Reports, P.O. Box 1051, STN MAIN, Fort Erie ON L2A 6C7.

Contents

INTRODUCTION 1

ALLERGIES. 3

ARM, LEG, AND FOOT AILMENTS 5
    Office Visit: When your feet start to swell 11

ARTHRITIS AND JOINT AND MUSCLE DISORDERS 13
    Office Visit: A bout of gout 17

ASTHMA AND LUNG PROBLEMS. 19
    Office Visit: When you can't catch a breath. 21

BACK PAIN. 24

BLADDER AND URINARY PROBLEMS 27

BLOOD PRESSURE 29

BONE HEALTH 33
    Office Visit: When it's not quite osteoporosis 36

CARDIOVASCULAR DISORDERS 38
    Office Visit: A preventable cause of stroke. 42
    Office Visit: Heart attack on a platter .44

CHOLESTEROL. 47

COLON AND RECTAL COMPLAINTS 53

CYSTS, LUMPS, AND TUMORS 57

DENTAL CARE 59

Office Visit: Is that dental X-ray necessary? 62

DIABETES 65
    Office Visit: The other diabetes. 66

DIET AND NUTRITION. 68

DOCTORS 90
    Office Visit: Your symptoms: Say what you mean. 91
    Office Visit: How to haggle with your doctor 93
    Office Visit: Six things to do in a doctor's waiting room 95

EAR PROBLEMS 98

EYE CARE. 100
    Office Visit: No silver bullet for dry-eye syndrome 105

EXERCISE AND FITNESS. 108

HAIR CARE 117

HEADACHES 120
    Office Visit: Tracking down migraine triggers 122
HEALTH FEARS AND RISKS 125
    Office Visit: Lyme disease: Beyond the rash 129
HEARTBURN 132
LIVER DISORDERS 134
MEDICAL PROCEDURES 135
    Office Visit: Is that stress test really necessary? 138
MEDICATIONS 140
MEN'S HEALTH . . . . : . 144
NEUROLOGICAL PROBLEMS 149
    Office Visit: The (not so) benign tremor 151
    Office Visit: When nerves go on strike 154
    Office Visit: When you hit your head 156
NOSE, MOUTH, AND THROAT DISORDERS 159
    Office Visit: Sore throat? Hold the antibiotics 160
    Office Visit: A tough one to swallow 168
PARENTING AND PREGNANCY 171
RESPIRATORY INFECTIONS 173
SKIN CARE 174
    Office Visit: To scratch an itch 182
STOMACH AILMENTS 185
    Office Visit: Intestinal gas: A right of passage? 189
    Office Visit: When the going gets tough 191
THE THYROID 194
    Office Visit: The dangers of silent thyroid disease 195
VACCINES 198
    Office Visit: Why we need vaccines 202
VITAMINS AND SUPPLEMENTS 204
    Office Visit: Vitamin B12: Panacea or placebo? 207
    Office Visit: The perils of dietary supplements 210
WATER: DIET AND SAFETY 213
WEIGHT CONTROL 215
    Office Visit: Explaining unexplained weight loss 216
WOMEN'S HEALTH 221

INDEX 226

Preface

Consumer Reports Best of Health is published by Consumer Reports, the nonprofit organization that publishes *Consumer Reports on Health*, a monthly newsletter on nutrition, fitness, and medical matters, and *Consumer Reports*, the monthly magazine best known for test reports, product Ratings, and buying guidance. *Consumer Reports* is also a comprehensive source of unbiased advice about products and services, personal finance, health and nutrition, and other consumer concerns. Since 1936, our mission has been to test products, inform the public, and protect consumers. Our income is derived solely from the sale of *Consumer Reports* magazine and our other publications and services, and from nonrestrictive, noncommercial contributions, grants, and fees. We buy all the products we test. We accept no ads from companies, nor do we let any company use our reports or Ratings for commercial purposes.

SERVICES FROM CONSUMER REPORTS

CONSUMER REPORTS. Published monthly, *Consumer Reports* magazine provides impartial information on brand-name products, services, health, and personal finance. To subscribe (13 issues, including the annual buying guide, $29), write to us at our Customer Service Department, P.O. Box 2109, Harlan, Iowa 51593-0298.

CONSUMER REPORTS ON HEALTH. Monthly newsletter offering solid, scientific research translated into simple, do-able, how-to advice that makes good health easy. Subscription rate: $24 for 1 year (12 issues). Phone orders call: 800-234-2188.

CONSUMER REPORTS MONEY ADVISER. Monthly newsletter offering financial advice and money-saving tips to help you make personal financial decisions with confidence. Subscription rate: $29 for 1 year (12 issues). To subscribe, call our service line: 800-234-1970.

SHOP SMART. Published 10 times per year, *ShopSmart* magazine is your best source for bargains and shopping tips. U.S. only: $34.95 for 1 year (10 issues). To subscribe, call 866-428-5812.

CONSUMER REPORTS SPECIAL PUBLICATIONS. We publish a series of specialty buying guides on cars, computers, and products for the home, as well as books on finance, drugs, and other issues of consumer concern. Consumer Reports Special Publications are available on newsstands and in bookstores, or through our Web store (www.ConsumerReports.org/books).

CONSUMER REPORTS WEB SITES. ConsumerReports.org offers convenient access to our product information and advice. Site subscribers pay $6.95 a month or $30 a year ($20 for *Consumer Reports* subscribers) for unlimited use of searchable ratings, recommendations, and consumer advice.

Introduction

Since its launch in 1989, a popular feature in the *Consumer Reports on Health* newsletter is "On Your Mind," a column in which the editors answer questions from readers on a wide variety of health topics. Most of the contents of *The Best of Health* have been drawn from this source.

The Best of Health also includes many "Office Visit" columns, a regular feature in *Consumer Reports on Health*, by Marvin M. Lipman, M.D., Consumers Union's chief medical adviser. These discussions, highly readable and full of practical advice, cover a wide range of health problems. The case histories are taken directly from Dr. Lipman's own medical practice. Orly Avitzur, M.D., Medical Editor, joins the discussion with an "Office Visit" on 95, 122, and 156. And guest columnists R. Linsy Farris, M.D., M.P.H., and John Santa M.D., M.P.H., weigh in on pages 105 and 93, respectively. And our dental expert, Jay Friedman, D.D.S., M.P.H. offers his insights on dental X-rays on page 62.

The Best of Health is easy to use. Each major topic is listed alphabetically, with specific problems arranged under the appropriate heading. Following many of the main questions and answers are "Office Visit" columns that discuss the same topic from a different angle and in greater detail.

Simply check the table of contents or consult the index to find the subjects that interest you. You're bound to find some questions (and answers) or some health-topic discussions that affect you, a family member, or a friend. Or read the book straight through. Once you get started, *The Best of Health* is hard to put down.

We think you'll find this book enlightening, entertaining, and a valuable source of reliable medical information. All the information has been carefully checked for accuracy and currency.

Allergies

DUST-MITE CONTROL

Q *Both my wife and I are allergic to dust mites and have tried the recommended step of washing our bedding every two weeks in hot water. However, hot water shrinks and ruins many items like comforters, blankets, and flannel sheets. A product called De-Mite, a laundry additive, claims to eliminate dust mites, even in cold water. Does this product really work? Also, do the carpet sprays and powders effectively "neutralize" dust mites and their allergens?*

A The active ingredient in *De-Mite,* benzyl benzoate, does indeed effectively kill dust mites when added to laundry detergent in a cool-water wash (2 tablespoons per load). One study found that ordinary detergent with a benzyl benzoate additive eliminated 99.8 percent of dust mites from textiles—compared with a 70.4 percent reduction without the additive—when used with 86°F/30°C wash water. Some carpet treatments also use benzyl benzoate, while others contain tannic acid. Both have been shown to neutralize dust-mite allergens for a few months. However, if you have wall-to-wall carpets, your best bet is to completely remove them from the house.

LESS ALLERGENIC FLOWERS

Q *Flowers seem to aggravate my allergies. Are certain types less likely to do that?*

A Yes. The key is the flowers' aroma, since you're probably reacting to their smell, not their pollen. (Unlike grass pollen and most tree pollens, flower pollens seldom get into the air;

they're actually spread mainly by insects and animals rather than wind.) So try to choose relatively low-scent flowers, such as crocuses, daffodils, daisies, certain roses, and tulips.

ALLERGY SHOTS

Q I've been taking immunotherapy shots to quell allergies for a year, but my allergist says I still need more shots. Is that normal?

A Yes. The shots can provide long-term relief from certain allergies by exposing the body to gradually increasing doses of the triggering substance, notably plant pollens, dust mites, and insect venom. But the process takes time: After about four months of weekly or biweekly injections, you'll need monthly booster shots for three to five years. Partly because of that inconvenience, the shots are generally recommended only when other strategies, such as antihistamine drugs or dust-mite covers on mattresses, bedding, and sofas, have failed to adequately control symptoms.

ELIMINATING ALLERGENS

Q In your recent article on food allergies, you said that alcohol sanitizers don't effectively remove allergens. Why?

A Alcohol-based hand sanitizers kill bacteria; they don't destroy food proteins, which cause food allergies. In a study of 12 people at Johns Hopkins University, alcohol sanitizers were no better than plain water at removing peanut residue from participants' hands. Washing with soap and water or using wipes were the most effective methods.

ANTIHISTAMINES IN ADVANCE?

Q *Should antihistamines be taken prior to allergy season, before symptoms develop, in order to build up immunity against the onslaught of allergens?*

A No. Antihistamines have no such "priming" effect. They help to combat allergic symptoms only when allergens (allergy-inducing substances) are present.

Arm, leg, and foot ailments

STUB OUT TOENAIL FUNGUS?

Q *Is there any cure for the fungus that is deforming my toenail?*

A There are two popular home and over-the-counter remedies: water-diluted vinegar foot soaks and *Vicks VapoRub*. We think that *VapoRub*—which contains eucalyptus, menthol, camphor, and other oils—may be worth a try since it is relatively cheap and nontoxic.

Two prescription oral antifungal drugs, terbinafine (*Lamisil* and generic) and itraconazole (*Sporanox* and generic), have been in use for several years and have been shown to be effective in up to 50 percent of takers. Monitoring is necessary, since either can be toxic to the liver. A three-month course of treatment can run up to several hundred dollars, not including doctor visits and tests. Bear in mind that there is no medicine that is effective or safe for everyone.

Ciclopirox (*Penlac Nail Lacquer* and generic) is a less effective paint-on medication. It has to be applied daily for at least four months, often longer. Laser treatment recently arrived on the scene, and a single treatment, usually by a podiatrist, may be effective nearly 90 percent of the time, but at around $1,200 a pop.

ATHLETE'S AGGRAVATION

Q *I'm worried about getting athlete's foot from my gym. Are there steps I can take to prevent it?*

A Yes. Athlete's foot is a contagious fungal infection that thrives in damp, warm places. It causes cracked, itchy skin and can lead to thickened, discolored toenails. To minimize your risk, wear flip-flops or sandals in locker rooms or public showers, and dry your feet completely after they get wet, especially between your toes. Avoid sharing towels. Cover any cuts or scrapes on your feet until they heal. Wear clean socks and well-ventilated shoes, and let shoes air out for a day between workouts. For people at high risk of athlete's foot, regular use of a powder containing aluminum chloride (an antiperspirant) can help prevent infection, and the powder or an antifungal cream such as terbinafine *(Lamisil AT* and generic) might prevent reinfection.

NUMB HAND AND ARM

Q *I experience recurring numbness during the day or night, especially in two fingers of the right hand. And I often wake up with my entire left arm numb and cold. What's the problem?*

A Your favorite sleeping position—like placing your hand under your pillow—could be numbing your left arm by putting pressure on a nerve. If so, feeling should return soon after you wake up and change position. Daytime numbness in your other hand most likely reflects a pinched nerve in your neck. Ask your doctor about being evaluated for disorders such as disk disease or arthritis of the neck, both of which are usually treatable with exercise, drugs, or, as a last resort, surgery.

COLD HANDS AND FEET

Q *My hands and feet are always cold. Does that signal some physical disorder?*

A Usually not. Some people have cold extremities for no apparent reason. In others, the coldness stems from anxiety or stress. It's also a side effect of certain drugs, notably beta-blockers and many migraine-fighting drugs. However, if your fingers or toes temporarily turn white, the coldness is probably caused by Raynaud's disease, a common condition that impairs circulation to the extremities. Severe cases can lead to fingertip ulceration. Raynaud's can occasionally signal a more serious disease, such as scleroderma or lupus. Treatment includes stopping smoking, keeping the hands and feet warm, and if necessary, taking blood-vessel-dilating ACE inhibitors or calcium-channel blockers.

CORN-REMOVAL CONCERNS

Q *A podiatrist told me that the acid in a medicated corn-removal pad can eat away not only the corn but also healthy skin, possibly causing infection. Is that true?*

A Yes. That's why the medicated pads should be small enough that they touch only the corn—a buildup of thick, hardened skin—not the surrounding area. Don't wear them longer than 48 hours, and check periodically to make sure the pad hasn't shifted off the corn. Never use pads on skin that is irritated or infected, and avoid them if you have diabetes or poor circulation, both of which increase the chance of irritation and infection. If you have none of those conditions and want an alternative to pads, try gently rubbing the corn with a callus file or pumice stone, available at drugstores, or even with a rough towel. Pharmacies also sell nonmedicated cushions, gel toe sleeves, and lambswool padding, which can ease discomfort when you walk. Wearing properly fitted shoes and having foot deformities treated can keep corns from developing or returning.

SLEEPY ARM

Q *I generally sleep on my side and often wake up with an arm that is numb. Is that dangerous?*

A Probably not. Temporary paresthesia—the "pins and needles" feeling you get when a limb goes numb—is usually a result of putting sustained pressure on a nerve. Sensation usually returns to the limb quickly once the pressure is removed, and there's generally no lasting effect. Arm numbness after sleeping on your side can be caused by the compression of spinal nerves in the neck or other nerves in the arm or shoulder. If you're experiencing chronic neck pain or stiffness, or if pain persists after the numbness in your arm subsides, it might be worth trying other sleeping positions as well as mentioning your concerns to your doctor.

WATERLOGGED LEGS

Q *I am a 75-year-old woman. Last year my feet and legs became so swollen that I couldn't get into my shoes. My doctor said I had "water retention" and gave me a seven-day supply of* Maxzide *(triamterene and hydrochlorothiazide), which eventually relieved the swelling. What causes water retention, and how can I avoid it?*

A There are several reasons for leg swelling. One of the most common is varicose veins, in which damage to valves in the large veins of the legs hinders the return of blood to the heart. Blood plasma, which is mostly water, pools in nearby tissue, causing swelling of the legs and feet. Excess dietary salt, sitting or standing for long periods, and hot weather can aggravate the swelling. Exercise such as walking or cycling helps. So does resting with your legs elevated. Water retention can also be caused by more serious problems, such as heart, liver, and kidney disorders. A medical checkup to rule those out would be wise.

FEET ON FIRE

Q *I have a severe burning feeling on the soles of both feet. My circulation is normal, and soaking and applying powders haven't helped. Could this be a symptom of a serious ailment?*

A A burning sensation on the soles of your feet can arise from any number of causes, from ill-fitting shoes to diabetes. The most serious cause is peripheral neuropathy—damage to the leg nerves—often from diabetes or alcoholism and less commonly from vitamin deficiencies or lead poisoning. A rare disorder called erythromelalgia increases blood flow to the hands and feet and can also produce a searing sensation.

Some people experience fiery feet because they're sensitive to a chemical in the inner lining of their shoes (particularly some types of athletic shoes). Try changing your footgear to see if the problem subsides. If not, see your physician to rule out medical causes.

VICKS ON FEET

Q *I got a chain e-mail message that claimed that putting* Vicks VapoRub *on your feet can help stop coughing. Is that true?*

A Probably not. *Vicks VapoRub* and similar products contain camphor and menthol, ingredients that are FDA-approved to help quell coughs when applied topically to the chest and neck. A long-standing Internet rumor holds that putting *Vicks* on children's feet and covering them with socks helps reduce coughing, and suggests the method works for adults, too. But there's no solid research to support that claim. And it's unsafe to use camphor on kids younger than 2.

TREATING SWOLLEN LEGS

Q *I've had lymphedema in both legs for 12 years, and my ability to walk has steadily worsened. My doctor's only recommendation is an extremity pump to pressurize a sleeve that covers each leg. Are there any other treatments?*

A Lymphedema is swelling of an arm or leg due to obstruction of the flow of lymph, a milky-looking body fluid. Leg swelling from lymphedema can be treated in several ways, but all treatments lose effectiveness over time. The "lymph pump" you describe can provide temporary relief early on, when fluid accumulation is less severe. The primary treatment for lymphedema remains the use of good elastic stockings. Various surgical procedures have been tried, generally with little lasting benefit.

✚ *Office* **Visit**

When your feet start to swell

SOME YEARS AGO, NEARING THE END OF A SIX-HOUR FLIGHT from New York to London, I found myself in a fix. I was unable to put my shoes back on. I had removed them soon after takeoff for comfort. During the flight I enjoyed several snack packages of pretzels and salted peanuts, and a meal (yes, airlines were serving them then) of spicy lasagna. At one point, I considered going for a walk but was dissuaded by the presence of two hefty fellows, both snoring loudly, between my window seat and the aisle. Resigned, I joined them in slumberland. Hours later, as the plane was nearing Heathrow, I discovered that my feet had swelled just enough to give me visions of roaming the airport in my socks. Were it not for a friendly flight attendant with a shoehorn, that vision might have become reality.

Swelling of the feet, ankles, and legs, or peripheral edema, is the reason for countless office visits each year. Since the causes are so numerous, that symptom also poses a diagnostic challenge to physicians. One way to understand edema is to consider why it doesn't happen all the time.

Edema fluid is a filtrate of blood plasma, the liquid that blood cells float around in, that seeps from the veins and into the tissues of the ankle and foot. Normally, edema doesn't form because 1) the hydrostatic pressure exerted against the walls of the veins isn't high enough to force the fluid out, and 2) large proteins in the blood, mainly albumin, exert osmotic pressure (the opposite of hydrostatic pressure) that prevents leakage from the veins. Anything that upsets the delicate balance between these two opposing pressures can result in the escape of fluid from the veins into the tissues.

Too much pressure

The causes of increased hydrostatic pressure are many and varied. One of the most common is varicose veins. Healthy veins have one-way valves that prevent blood from pooling in the legs and thus raising hydrostatic pressure. Heredity, pregnancy, inflammation, or a job that involves a lot of time on your feet (dentist, letter carrier, surgeon) can damage those valves. Another common cause of increased venous pressure is congestive heart failure, which causes blood to back up in the veins that return blood to the heart. In addition, any abdominal or pelvic mass, such as a tumor or fibroids, can impinge on veins, block the flow of blood toward the heart, and raise pressure in the leg veins.

Overexpansion of blood plasma is another way of raising hydrostatic pressure in the venous system. This happens with chronic kidney disease, which impairs the body's ability to excrete fluid. It can also result from the zealous use of intravenous fluids in some hospitalized patients. A commonly used class of medications known as nonsteroidal anti-inflammatory drugs (NSAIDs), such as ibuprofen *(Advil, Motrin,* and generic) and naproxen *(Aleve* and generic), reduce inflammation by interfering with production of a pro-inflammatory hormone called prostaglandin. Because prostaglandin helps excrete sodium, its absence causes sodium retention, and with it, water retention and blood-volume expansion. Other drugs that can cause volume expansion include two for diabetes—pioglitazone *(Actos)* and rosiglitazone *(Avandia)*—and one class of antihypertensives—calcium-channel blockers such as amlodipine *(Norvasc* and generic).

Too little pressure

The second of the two underlying causes of edema is a reduction in the osmotic pressure in the blood due to protein depletion. The poster child for this condition is the protein-starved victim with a potbelly and swollen legs in an otherwise emaciated body. In this country, edema due to protein depletion is most often seen with certain forms of kidney disease and liver failure.

Finally, some people can develop mild, transient edema without having a disease or taking edema-causing medication. It can happen during the second half of the menstrual cycle or during the third trimester of pregnancy (when it might signal the onset of pregnancy-induced hypertension). It can also happen to someone silly enough to consume massive amounts of salt-rich foods and remain glued to his seat on a plane in one position for hours on end.

Since that episode, I book aisle seats on long flights and bring my own low-sodium snacks for nourishment.

Arthritis and joint and muscle disorders

RAIN AND BONES

Q *Some people say they can tell when it's going to rain because they can "feel" it in their bones. Is this true?*

A Yes. Changes in the weather—including a fall in atmospheric pressure, which can signal rain—can alter the pressure in the space surrounding joints, sometimes enough to cause perceptible discomfort. The effect is especially painful for people with joint conditions such as rheumatoid arthritis, particularly when the weather changes suddenly. People with muscle inflammation or previous injuries may also suffer weather-related pain. An over-the-counter pain reliever such as acetaminophen (*Tylenol* and generic) or ibuprofen (*Advil* and generic), or using an ice pack for 15 to 20 minutes on sore areas might provide some relief. Gentle exercise and stretching might also help.

HEAT OR COLD FOR ARTHRITIS?

Q *Is it better to treat arthritis symptoms with heat or cold?*

A That depends on the symptoms. Cold reduces inflammation and swelling and relieves pain better than heat (though alternating between cold and heat provides greater relief for some people). But cold may increase joint stiffness. Heat relaxes muscles and tendons and promotes circulation, so it's the best choice for boosting the mobility of stiff joints. Finally, heat and cold can each help tame muscle spasms.

Whichever approach you choose, follow these precautions:

• Apply heat or cold for only 15 to 20 minutes at a time, letting the skin return to normal temperature before reapplying.

• Place a cloth or towel between your skin and the heating or cooling device.

• Stop immediately if your skin blisters or turns either dark red or spotty red and white.

Don't use heat or cold on damaged skin. And don't use them at all if you suffer from poor circulation, nerve damage, or a condition that may cause either of those problems, such as diabetes, Raynaud's disease, or vasculitis.

DISJOINTED FINGERS

Q *I recently dislocated a finger while carrying a heavy plastic shopping bag. What's the best way to treat it?*

A Dislocations occur when two bones normally connected by a flexible joint pop out of alignment. Fingers are the most common site for those injuries, since they're used so frequently and are relatively fragile. Your primary-care doctor can usually pop the bone back into place. As long as an X-ray shows no signs of fracture, a simple splint to allow healing of the stretched tendons is all that's needed.

RUB IT IN

Q *What is it about* Bengay *that helps relieve the pain of arthritis?*

A *Bengay,* like other muscle-ache and arthritis rubs, provides relief by acting as a counterirritant. It produces a mild local inflammation that crowds out pain messages from nearby muscles and joints. Arthritis rubs also create heat by increasing blood flow to the area; because of the risk of a burn, they should never be used together with a heating pad.

BURSITIS OF THE HIP

Q *How common is bursitis of the hip, and what can be done about it? I had my first siege 10 months ago, and although* Feldene *helped a lot, the bursitis has not disappeared entirely.*

A Although bursitis most often affects the shoulder, bursitis of the hip is also quite common. Knees and elbows are also vulnerable. At all those joints, tiny sacs called bursae cover the area where the tendon attaches to the bone. When a bursa becomes inflamed, often because of injury or overuse, the joint aches. Standard treatment consists of rest and oral anti-inflammatory medication such as naproxen (*Aleve, Naprosyn,* and generic). Sometimes injections of a corticosteroid drug directly into the bursa can be helpful. The inflammation and pain usually pass with time but can recur. In rare instances, surgery may be necessary.

MUSCLE CRAMPS

Q *As I've grown older, I've started getting muscle cramps. What can I do about them?*

A For most cramps, stretch. If a spasm strikes the calf (by far the most common cramp site), pull the front of the foot up toward the knee. Since cramps usually result from muscle fatigue, you may be able to prevent such spasms by gently stretching before you exercise your calves. Stretching before bedtime can also help prevent unexplained nighttime spasms.

If the cause isn't muscle fatigue, your physician may find other, possibly treatable causes. These can include circulatory problems, hyperventilation, an underactive thyroid, and low blood levels of calcium or (rarely) magnesium.

ARTHRITIS SUPPLEMENTS

Q *Can I buy glucosamine by itself—that is, when it's not combined with chondroitin?*

A Yes, but you should look for products that contain glucosamine sulfate, which has better supporting evidence than other forms, including glucosamine hydrochloride and N-acetylglucosamine. Some clinical trials have found that people with osteoarthritis who take glucosamine sulfate have slightly less joint pain and better function than those taking a placebo, though other trials have shown no benefit. Glucosamine may not be safe for people taking blood thinners.

✚ *Office* **Visit**

A bout of gout

"I DIDN'T KNOW THAT WOMEN COULD GET GOUT!" SAID THE 52-year-old financial adviser who limped into the office leaning on a crutch. I had mentioned that the two leading possible causes of her right-knee pain were an infection and gout. "I was fine yesterday and had only a little ache in the right knee when I went to bed," she told me. "I was awakened about 3 in the morning by the worst pain I've ever had. I couldn't bear the covers touching my knee, which was swollen, bright red, and hot to the touch." A quick consultation with a rheumatology colleague led to the removal of some clear, yellowish fluid from the knee joint. Microscopic examination of the fluid showed typical needlelike sodium-urate crystals. The diagnosis of gout was assured.

Charles Dickens's 1836 novel, *The Pickwick Papers*, established the image of a gout victim as a stout, middle-aged, pipe-smoking gentleman with a bandaged foot resting on a hassock and a glass of port within easy reach. While dietary excess and overindulgence in alcohol can indeed trigger the symptoms of gout, that 19th-century stereotype looked nothing like my slim, teetotaling female patient.

A common disease

Gout affects about 6.1 million adults in the U.S., and the number of cases is increasing. It tends to attack suddenly. The favored joint is the large one at the base of the great toe, though elbows, knees, and ankles are also vulnerable. The pain is excruciating, and anyone who can wait seven to 10 days for the attack to subside on its own has got to be a masochist. Repeated gout episodes can leave deposits of sodium-urate crystals (tophi) that cause joint enlargement and nodule formation in the arms and legs.

Three or four times more men than women develop gout, but the difference narrows with menopause, since estrogen promotes uric-acid excretion in the urine. And that simple chemical substance—uric acid—is the culprit.

Virtually all mammals are able to break down ingested protein into a harmless, easily excreted substance, allantoin, with the help of an enzyme, uricase. That enzyme completes the last step—the metabolism of uric acid to allantoin. Not so in humans and their cousins, the great apes, in whom the Darwinian evolutionary plan inexplicably saw fit to eliminate uricase so that protein metabolism ends with uric acid, which is hard for the body to get rid of.

Gout results when uric-acid crystals irritate a joint lining and cause inflammation. The causes for this uric-acid buildup include eating too many protein-rich foods (especially meat and seafood), drinking alcohol or soft drinks, and consuming food containing fructose. Those who drink large amounts of coffee, consume dairy products, or take vitamin C supplements tend to have lower rates of uric-acid production. But the main problem for most people might be simply an inherited tendency for the kidneys to hold on to uric acid.

Treatment is effective

Once gout is diagnosed, treatment is simple. The condition responds as if by magic to anti-inflammatory medication (so if you're the doctor, the patient becomes your friend for life). Corticosteroids (prednisone, prednisolone) and nonsteroidals (ibuprofen, naproxen) in full anti-inflammatory doses are now the treatments of choice. Colchicine, an inexpensive and popular gout remedy known since 1820, was, oddly, not approved by the Food and Drug Administration until 2009. It is now available only as a relatively expensive brand-name product, *Colcrys*, which has been downgraded to a second-line drug, probably because it frequently causes diarrhea.

For long-term treatment to prevent episodes of acute gout as well as the formation of tophi and uric-acid kidney stones, the preferred medicine is allopurinol (*Zyloprim* and generic). An expensive alternative, febuxostat (*Uloric*), was approved in 2009. Generic probenecid, a treatment alternative, lowers blood uric acid by increasing its excretion in the urine.

I put the financial adviser on a weeklong regimen of prednisone. Her knee was almost back to normal the day after she started the medication. Her blood uric-acid level, usually increased in people with gout, was borderline at the time of the attack. We are following it periodically, and I have advised her to switch to a low-protein diet with increased dairy intake. Her chances of having a second attack within the next year are about 60 percent. We'll keep our fingers crossed.

Asthma and lung problems

ASTHMA AND GAS STOVES

Q I understand that using a wood-burning fireplace or stove can aggravate asthma and allergies. Is that also true of appliances that use gas logs?

A Like woodstoves, all gas-burning appliances emit several invisible combustion byproducts, such as carbon monoxide and nitrous oxides, some of which can irritate the lungs. In one study of 539 adults with asthma, the researchers found that those who used gas stoves daily were twice as likely to suffer severe asthma attacks as those who never used such appliances. Since the offending pollutants are too small to be filtered out of the air, the only way to reduce or eliminate them is to improve the ventilation or give up the gas.

BLOOD CLOTS IN THE LUNG

Q *Four weeks after having a hysterectomy, my 62-year-old mother died suddenly because of pulmonary emboli, or blood clots in her lung. Should my sisters and I worry that this could happen to us after surgery?*

A That depends. Susceptibility to pulmonary embolism, which generally develops only after surgery or prolonged bed rest, is not inherited directly. However, two risk factors for the condition—obesity and severe varicose veins—do run in families. Other risk factors include heart failure, certain cancers, a history of phlebitis (inflamed veins), and long rides in trains and airplanes. People predisposed to pulmonary embolism may receive anticlotting medication after they've undergone abdominal, pelvic, or certain orthopedic operations—or if they'll be bedridden for a long time or taking a long flight.

GOOD MOVES FOR ASTHMATICS

Q *I'm considering a change of climate to help relieve my asthma. I've heard that the dry air of the desert Southwest is beneficial, but also that salty sea air can help. Can you clear up this contradiction?*

A The best locale for asthma sufferers is one that's free of pollutants, airborne allergens, and frigid weather. Traditionally, asthmatics migrated to Arizona for its warm, dry climate, although the benefit came primarily from cleaner air and lower pollen counts. As Arizona cities have grown, however, the environment there has become less favorable for asthmatics. Sea air has no effect on asthma.

✚ *Office* **Visit**

When you can't catch a breath

A LONGTIME FRIEND OF MINE, AGE 82, WAS ALWAYS KNOWN TO be in excellent health. But she complained that for the past few weeks she had trouble breathing. She was fine at rest but became short of breath with the least exertion. Normally, she could climb several flights of stairs with ease. Now, she could barely negotiate one flight—one step at a time—and became breathless after just a minute of walking. She said she had no associated symptoms, such as fever, chest pain, cough, leg swelling, or wheezing. She hadn't smoked since her college days. Her exam, chest X-ray, and routine lab tests were normal.

Understanding breathlessness

Seeing, smelling, swallowing, walking, and even digesting are activities that we don't think much about until a cataract, cold, strep throat, arthritic knee, or heartburn intervene. Then what was taken for granted suddenly becomes a focus of attention.

Breathing is one such unconscious activity. Most of us do it automatically at least 20,000 times a day. Its sole purpose is to supply the body with oxygen and rid it of carbon dioxide. If anything interferes with that exchange of gases, causing a deficit of oxygen or a surplus of carbon dioxide, the breathing rate will automatically increase to compensate. You will perceive that as shortness of breath or, in medicalese, dyspnea.

The mechanics of normal breathing involve not only the heart and lungs but also the muscles of the chest wall and the nervous system, so the causes of dyspnea are many. Nevertheless, with proper evaluation, the diagnosis is apparent about two-thirds of the time. Risk factors such as smoking, chronic exposure to irritating chemicals, or the use of certain medication, notably beta-blockers (such as atenolol or metoprolol), can be important clues. Signs and symptoms such as cough, bloody or colored sputum, wheezing, chills, fever, chest pain, ankle swelling, and heartburn are giveaways for diagnoses such as pneumonia, asthma, pulmonary embolism, heart failure, and acid reflux. Anemia, a deficiency of oxygen-carrying red blood cells, also commonly produces dyspnea on exertion.

But not all shortness of breath is caused by disease. When we exercise, our muscles require more oxygen than they do when we are at rest. Therefore our breathing rate increases and our heart beats faster to satisfy that need. Visitors to high altitudes, where the oxygen content of the air is lower than what they're used to, often find breathing difficult. People who live in such regions become acclimated when their red blood cell count increases, thereby improving their body's oxygen content.

And what pregnant woman hasn't complained of shortness of breath from respiratory stress caused by her swollen belly and increased weight? Chronic anxiety can produce a type of air hunger characterized by "sighing respirations," often described as being "unable to get on top of a breath." This differs from the hyperventilation episodes that are more likely associated with acute anxiety, and which result in intense tingling of the extremities, faintness, and occasionally loss of consciousness.

Problem solved

My friend's shortness of breath on exertion was a puzzle—that is, until I asked her to walk around my office building and checked her oxygen level and pulse rate before and after that mild exercise. Imagine my surprise when her pulse rate dropped instead of increasing as expected. An electrocardiogram showed that with exercise, each electrical impulse, initiated in an upper heart chamber, had an increasingly difficult time activating the lower heart chambers to cause a heartbeat. This condition is called heart block, and sometimes, as in her case, occurs only upon physical exertion. It prevented the increase in heart rate required to supply her tissues with oxygen, which in turn caused her breathing to speed up in an effort to make up the deficit. My cardiologist colleague suggested implanting a permanent cardiac pacemaker, which was done a few days later and solved the problem immediately. She has resumed her usual activities and continues to do well. Our attempts to find a cause for the heart block came up empty.

ONE TOO MANY

Q *I live a healthy lifestyle except for one vice: I smoke one cigarette a day. Do my otherwise healthful habits negate the risks?*

A Sorry, but no. Even "light" smoking (one to four cigarettes a day) increases the risk of heart disease and premature death in men and women, and it increases the risk of lung cancer in women, evidence shows. While less smoking is certainly better than more, strong research has found that it's no match for quitting. In a study involving more than 100,000 people, for example, the number of years spent smoking increased the risk of death from lung cancer more than the number of cigarettes smoked each day. The good news is that the less you smoke, the easier it is to stop. If you need help, the American Cancer Society offers free information about smoking cessation at 800-ACS-2345 or *www.cancer.org*.

Back pain

DISK DECISION

Q *Because of a herniated disk, I've been suffering from lower-back pain that radiates to my leg. Is surgery usually necessary, or could other treatment relieve the pain?*

A Conservative treatment, including physical therapy and anti-inflammatory drugs, is often successful in relieving pain from a herniated, or "slipped," disk. Unless the pain or numbness is severe or nerve function is impaired to the point of weakness of your leg muscles, you should try those alternatives for two to three months before resorting to more invasive techniques.

SPINAL SURGERY

Q *My doctor suggested minimally invasive surgery for my back pain. Is it worth trying?*

A Only as a last resort. Minimally invasive decompression surgery uses smaller incisions than the standard operation, which involves slicing through the muscles and bones of the lower back to relieve pressure on nerves from slipped disks or other causes. But in a 2008 *Consumer Reports* survey of some 1,000 readers who underwent back surgery, nearly half said that recovery was longer and more painful than expected. And most back pain resolves on its own in about six weeks. When it doesn't, acupuncture, chiropractic care, or exercise often help. So consider surgery only if other options have failed and you've received a second opinion.

PUSH-UPS AND BAD BACKS

Q *I've read that anyone with a "bad back" should not do push-ups. I've never experienced any back problems that I could attribute to push-ups, but now I am concerned. Please elaborate.*

A Done correctly, push-ups shouldn't harm your back at all. The key is to keep your upper body straight as you push up, whether pivoting from your toes (the classic position) or from your knees (the "modified" push-up). If you arch your back, you'll strain it. That's a common mistake, so people who have had back problems should probably skip push-ups.

INVERSION FOR BACK PAIN

Q *I'm hearing a lot lately about inversion tables. Do they work for back pain?*

A Probably not. Inversion tables are a form of traction therapy, which stretches the spine to theoretically increase space between vertebrae and reduce pressure on the back's disks. Inversion therapy involves lying at an incline with your head below your feet, and sometimes completely upside down. There's little or no evidence to support traction in general. Any benefits appear to be short-lived, and in some cases it might lead to increased pain. Lying in an inverted position can also drive up blood pressure. And several inversion products have been recalled for equipment failure that could lead to falls.

LUMBAR DECOMPRESSION

Q *I recently heard about a treatment called nonsurgical lumbar decompression. Can it help treat my lower-back pain?*

A There's not enough evidence to say. A procedure called vertebral axial decompression, or VAX-D, is offered at some spinal centers. It entails lying face-down on a special table that alternately pulls the lower body away from the upper body, then releases it, which purportedly relieves pain by decreasing pressure on the intervertebral disks. But the few studies we could find on it were small and often uncontrolled, and focused only on certain kinds of back pain, including herniated disks and trapped nerves. VAX-D isn't recommended for spinal stenosis, or narrowing of the spinal column. And most insurers don't cover the treatment, which can cost several thousand dollars.

SPINAL X-RAY RISKS

Q *In search of a diagnosis for my persistent low-back pain, my doctor recently ordered several X-rays of my spine. Do multiple X-rays increase my risk of developing cancer?*

A Yes. While nearly all X-rays expose you to radiation that increases your cancer risk, a low-back X-ray can expose you to relatively high doses. Moreover, those tests are often unnecessary, since nearly all low-back pain stems from muscles, ligaments, and nerves, which don't appear on X-rays. And most low-back pain eventually resolves on its own with simple self-help measures, including mild painkillers and cold packs. In general, agree to imaging tests only if the pain doesn't respond to self-help methods or physical therapy and lasts for more than a month, or if you also have any of the following: leg weakness; pain radiating from the buttock to the thigh, knee, or lower leg; a history of osteoporosis, or a recent fall or accident; fever, night sweats, or unexplained weight loss; or a history of cancer or incontinence.

Bladder and urinary problems

LONG-TERM DIURETICS

Q *I take a diuretic medication every day. Does the drug lose its effectiveness or cause any harm when taken for many years?*

A No. Diuretics (drugs that increase urine output) are an effective long-term therapy for hypertension and other disorders. Long-term use doesn't cause harm, although it can result in a low blood-potassium level, which can damage the kidneys.

WHEN YOU GOTTA GO, PART 1

Q *Your recent story about treatments for overactive bladder didn't mention underlying conditions that could cause bladder symptoms. Aren't there some?*

A Yes, many. An overactive bladder is characterized by frequent, overwhelming urges to urinate even if you've just gone to the bathroom, often accompanied by urine leakage if you don't get there in time. While its cause is unknown, a host of other conditions can produce similar symptoms, particularly urinary frequency, by irritating the bladder or interfering with the nerves or muscles involved in urination. Those include urinary-tract infections, interstitial cystitis, bladder stones, enlargement or infection of the prostate, spinal-cord tumors, stroke, Parkinson's disease, multiple sclerosis, and diabetes. Several drugs can have similar effects, most notably blood-pressure medications. If you suffer from symptoms of an overactive bladder, talk to your doctor about whether such drugs or conditions could be causing them.

WHEN YOU GOTTA GO, PART 2

Q *Frequent urination is considered a symptom of various conditions, including diabetes. But what qualifies as "frequent"?*

A In short, it's a level that's unusually frequent for you. Normal urinary frequency depends on many factors, including your bladder capacity, level of urinary control, and liquid intake. If you drink liquids often or in large amounts, then it's normal and healthy to urinate frequently. Alcohol, caffeine, and acidic foods can increase urinary frequency, as can certain drugs, namely diuretics. In general, talk with your doctor if you're passing very large volumes of urine, the frequency has increased with no identifiable cause (such as consuming more caffeine or changes in medication), or you have an increased urgency, possibly accompanied by bladder pain.

RESTLESS NIGHTS

Q *For the past few years, an aching fullness in my bladder has prompted me to get up three to four times a night to urinate. I do not experience the problem during the day. I am 25 years old, female, and otherwise in good health. Do I need to see a doctor?*

A Not necessarily. First, try drinking less fluid during the evening. In particular, refrain from alcohol and caffeine, which are diuretics. But if those simple measures don't work, see your doctor. Your "nocturia" could be due to an enlarged pelvic structure pressing on the bladder when you lie down, the nighttime release of daytime water retention, or a kidney disorder.

PELVIC EXERCISES

Q *I read that pelvic-floor contractions might help treat an overactive bladder and impotence. How does one do these?*

A The exercises, known as "Kegels," involve contracting and relaxing the pelvic-floor muscles that control your urine stream. To do them, squeeze the muscles as if you were trying to stop urinating; hold, then relax. Practice doing short ones lasting 2 seconds, and longer ones lasting 5 to 10 seconds. Try for 40 to 50 of each type a day, either all at once or in sets of 10 repetitions.

Blood pressure

BLOOD-PRESSURE FLUCTUATION

Q *Is it normal for blood pressure to fluctuate throughout the day?*

A Yes. Blood pressure—particularly the systolic pressure (upper number)—rises and falls throughout the day in response to what you're doing, feeling, and thinking. Caffeine, exercise, smoking, and stress temporarily increase blood pressure, while meditation and other calming activities, such as yoga, typically lower it. In a healthy person, blood pressure should also follow a certain daily rhythm, peaking in the morning, slowly declining in the afternoon and evening, falling even lower during the night, and again rising to greet the dawn. Blood pressure that doesn't follow that pattern could be an early warning sign of cardiovascular disease, which is why it's important for people monitoring their blood pressure at home to take several readings a day at the same times.

WHEN TO CHECK BLOOD PRESSURE

Q *I have hypertension. What's the best time of day to check my pressure?*

A Measure it at various times to determine when it's typically highest, then check it at that time each day; that provides the best information about possibly worrisome elevations. But also measure your blood pressure if you experience symptoms such as lightheadness, which might stem from too much antihypertensive medication. To ensure reliable results, rest your arm in the same position when taking a reading, and wait at least a half-hour after exercising or consuming caffeine, which can increase your pressure, or after eating, which can lower it.

BALANCING POTASSIUM NEEDS

Q *I have read that it's important to have 4,000 to 5,000 milligrams of potassium daily, mainly to keep blood pressure down. We regularly eat bananas and have a daily glass of orange juice, but those foods total only about 800 milligrams. My husband and I are in our mid-60s, and he is taking Prinivil for high blood pressure (mine is low). Should we strive to meet that potassium guideline?*

A Potassium has been shown to modestly reduce blood pressure, but that doesn't mean that more is better for everyone. Your husband, for instance, shouldn't increase his potassium intake as long as he is taking lisinopril (*Prinivil* and generic). Like all the blood-pressure drugs known as ACE inhibitors, lisinopril has a tendency to cause the kidneys to retain potassium. As for yourself, you can easily get all the potassium you need through a diet that contains plenty of fruits, vegetables, and dairy products. Orange juice (503 milligrams per cup) and bananas (451 milligrams each) are just a start. A single baked potato with skin contains 844 milligrams; a half-cup of cooked spinach, 420 milligrams; a cup of low-fat plain yogurt, 531 milligrams.

YO-YO BLOOD PRESSURE

Q My blood pressure bounces up and down from day to day, ranging from as high as 180/98 to as low as 107/61. I've been taking blood-pressure medication for years, but this fluctuation is relatively new, and nothing seems to help. Can you offer any suggestions?

A Ask your doctor about taking a 24-hour urine test to screen for an adrenaline-producing tumor called a pheochromocytoma. That treatable condition can cause wildly fluctuating blood pressure. A more common cause is nerve inflammation due to diabetes.

THE OTHER HYPERTENSION

Q What would cause an increase in a 70-year-old's systolic, or upper, blood-pressure reading while the diastolic pressure remains normal? How serious a problem is this?

A The stiffening of the arteries that typically occurs with advancing age can cause systolic blood pressure (the pressure in the arteries when the heart contracts) to rise above normal without affecting diastolic pressure (the pressure between contractions). An overactive thyroid or anemia can often produce the same effect. Temporary systolic blood-pressure hikes may result from exercise, stress, or excitement.

Until recently, doctors paid little attention to systolic blood pressure. But several studies have now clearly shown that for middle-aged and older people, any increase in systolic blood pressure over 140 mm Hg definitely needs to be controlled.

HEAT AND BLOOD PRESSURE

Q *Does using a* Jacuzzi *or sauna elevate blood pressure in people who already have hypertension?*

A No. In fact, high ambient temperature typically causes blood pressure to drop as blood vessels dilate in order to keep body temperature constant. That drop in blood pressure can cause you to faint, especially if you're already taking antihypertensive medication.

LOW BLOOD PRESSURE

Q *My blood pressure is naturally very low, though it doesn't seem to cause any symptoms. Is it possible to have low blood pressure that is too low?*

A Low blood pressure is defined as a systolic (upper reading) of 100 millimeters of mercury or less.

If no underlying cause is found and you have no symptoms, you needn't worry. In fact, people with naturally low blood pressure tend to live longer than people with "normal" pressure.

But if low blood pressure causes bothersome symptoms such as frequent or severe dizziness, or fainting when you stand up or have been standing for an extended period, then you might need to boost your pressure by wearing pressure stockings, consuming more salt, or taking a drug that raises your blood pressure. You should also check that your doctor has ruled out any underlying diseases that might cause low pressure, including diabetes or adrenal sufficiency.

Bone health

HEIGHT LOSS

Q *I'm 84 and have lost several inches from my 5-foot-11-inch frame. Is this normal? Is there anything I can do?*

A Yes and probably. As you age, the spongy disks between the vertebrae in the spine dry out and thin. If you have a bone-weakening condition such as osteoporosis, you may also experience spinal compression fractures—tiny, often imperceptible breaks in the vertebrae. Both can shorten the spine and thus your height. By age 80, women lose an average of about 3 inches in height, according to one large study; men lose about 2 inches. You can help minimize the loss by getting adequate calcium and vitamin D, and taking a bone-building drug such as alendronate (*Fosamax* and generic) if you have osteoporosis. Regular strength training and weight-bearing exercise such as walking can help maintain height by strengthening the skeleton. In severe cases where vertebral fractures have led to chronic back pain, stooped posture, or both, surgery may partly restore lost height and relieve discomfort.

TEA AND CALCIUM ABSORPTION

Q *I'm an avid tea drinker who's at risk for developing osteoporosis. I take calcium pills, but I've heard tea is high in oxalate, which blocks calcium absorption. Should I up my calcium dosage?*

A Probably not. Oxalate, a naturally occurring chemical in many foods, can significantly reduce the body's calcium absorption—but only from the same food, such as spinach and rhubarb, that contains the oxalate. There is no calcium in tea. And tea's oxalate won't significantly affect the absorption of calcium from supplements or other beverages or foods, even if they're consumed at the same time. In fact, two recent studies found that tea drinkers had stronger bones than nondrinkers, possibly because of the protective effects of flavonoids and fluoride in tea. Although calcium and oxalates can combine to form kidney stones, that condition tends to occur only if you consume lots of oxalate and not enough calcium. And some evidence suggests tea may help block stone development in other ways.

TUMS FOR THE BONES

My doctor told me to take Tums, *which is calcium carbonate, as an inexpensive alternative to calcium pills. However, the bottle warns against taking the maximum dose for more than two weeks. Is it safe to take* Tums *indefinitely?*

Yes, if you're just taking the modest dose needed as a supplement. The warning on the *Tums* bottle refers to its use as an antacid: Prolonged need for antacids should be evaluated by a doctor. Moreover, large amounts of supplemental calcium—such as the maximum dosage of 16 tablets a day for indigestion—can cause constipation, abdominal pain, and kidney stones if taken over a long period.

LIQUID CALCIUM

Are liquid calcium supplements absorbed better than calcium pills?

Possibly. Liquid or chewable supplements give the body a head start on absorption because they're already broken down when they reach the stomach. If you prefer pills, calcium carbonate has the highest percentage of calcium and usually costs less. Pick products that bear the seal of the U.S. Pharmacopeia (USP), which ensures they've been tested for purity and potency. You can also check your supplement's solubility by putting it in a glass of vinegar for 30 minutes and stirring periodically. If it doesn't dissolve, it probably won't be absorbed well in your stomach.

TORTUROUS TAILBONE

Q *I've been suffering from coccydynia, or painful tailbone, for over a year. It started suddenly, for no apparent reason, and it makes sitting very painful. I've seen several doctors, but none have helped. Do you have any suggestions?*

A First, make sure your doctors have checked for rare tumors and infections in the lower back that can trigger similar symptoms. More often, the problem stems from sprained tailbone ligaments. While that's usually caused by a fall or by difficult delivery of a child, the physical stress of sitting can eventually cause similar damage if you're overweight. If not, the pain may stem from an otherwise benign bone growth on the end of the tailbone. Mild pain can usually be soothed by taking anti-inflammatory drugs such as aspirin or ibuprofen (*Advil, Motrin,* and generic), sitting erect, or sitting on a donut-shaped pillow. But severe pain like yours will probably require stronger treatment. A combination of massage (preceded by a local-anesthetic injection) plus corticosteroid injections usually pacifies the pain. If all else fails and you can't live with the pain, you might consider removal of the entire tailbone, though the procedure is still fairly controversial, and full recovery can take up to a year.

✚ *Office* Visit

When it's not quite osteoporosis

A FEW YEARS AGO A 58-YEAR-OLD RETIRED HIGH SCHOOL teacher asked me if she *really* had to take *Fosamax* (alendronate), the bone-building drug prescribed by her gynecologist. A bone-density test done because she was six years postmenopausal found that she had what was then called osteopenia. She was leery of the possible side effects of *Fosamax*—including heartburn and jawbone weakening—and in no mood to commit to taking an expensive pill once a week for the next 5 to 10 years. She was neither a smoker nor a drinker, and had never broken so much as a toe. Her mother was alive and well and in her 80s.

Mind your T's and Z's

Osteoporosis (brittle-bone disease) is an important cause of fractures, pain, disability, and sometimes death in older women and, to a lesser extent, in older men. So doing everything possible to prevent it makes perfect sense. In lower-tech times, the only way to diagnose the condition was after a fracture or with an X-ray. The problem was that by the time bone had thinned enough to show up on an X-ray, full-blown osteoporosis had already developed.

In the late 1980s, the advent of bone mineral densitometry measured by dual-energy X-ray absorptiometry (DEXA) enabled clinicians to assess bone density with precision. This advance quickly resulted in the creation of a new "pre-osteoporosis" diagnostic category then called osteopenia (though now referred to as low bone density), which literally means "less bone."

A DEXA scan measures the patient's bone-calcium content, or bone density, at several sites (the lower spine, the hip, and, usually, the wrist). The score is then compared with the average score of 30-year-old women at the peak of their bone mass. The comparison is called the T score. The lower the T score, the higher the fracture risk.

A T score of minus 2.5 or worse indicates osteoporosis; a score ranging from minus 1 through minus 2.4 indicates low bone density. But the normal range in healthy 30-year-old women is from minus 2 to plus 2, so scores between minus 1 and minus 2 are technically normal. The Z score simply compares the patient with the average bone density of other women her age.

Several medications, including *Fosamax*, are approved not only to treat osteoporosis but also to prevent it. But while the use of those drugs has been shown to reduce the fracture rate in patients with osteoporosis, studies in patients with low bone density have been inconsistent or disappointing. Although the vast majority of postmenopausal women eventually develop some degree of low bone density, not all will go on to develop osteoporosis.

A question of risk

So, while in the past it may have been reasonable on the basis of established evidence for a physician to reach for the prescription pad if the patient has a T score of minus 2.5 SD or more, the decision to prescribe drugs for women with less-severe T scores should be weighted by the presence or absence of risk factors for fracture other than just their bone density.

The most important risk factors are a personal history of a fracture after age 50, a family history of fracture in a parent or sibling, body weight below 127 pounds, a current smoking habit, or a history of corticosteroid use for three months or more.

Additional risk factors are those that make any individual, with or without osteoporosis, more prone to falls. They include poor vision, dementia, neurological disorders such as stroke or Parkinson's disease, alcoholism, muscular problems, and the use of tranquilizers or sleeping pills.

In 2010, the World Health Organization developed a calculator known as FRAX, which is available online (www.shef.ac.uk/ FRAX), to aid in estimating fracture risk. The risk of fracture depends on how close you are to the cutoff for osteoporosis and how rapidly you're losing bone. FRAX takes these measurements and other mentioned risk factors into account.

The retired teacher had none of the previously mentioned risk factors. She had T scores of minus 1.7 SD in the lower spine, minus 1.6 SD in the hip, and minus 1.2 SD in the wrist. I told her to stop the *Fosamax* and increase her dietary calcium intake. In addition, although her vitamin D blood levels were normal, I advised her to take 800 international units a day to maintain those levels. She also enrolled in a program at a local gym, since weight-bearing exercise is an important stimulus to bone formation.

Two years later, I reviewed her bone-density measurements. None had deteriorated, and the lower spine had shown some improvement. She continues to exercise and take her supplements.

Cardiovascular disorders

RAPID HEARTBEAT

Q *My mother-in-law recently experienced a racing heart, about 130 beats per minute, throughout the night. Could that be serious?*

A Possibly, depending on the cause. It may have been a response to caffeine or pseudoephedrine (*Sudafed* and generic) taken too close to bedtime. But it could also stem from abnormalities of the nerve pathways that trigger the rhythmic contractions of the heart. The most common abnormalities involve the heart's upper chambers, or atria. Such atrial tachycardias, or rapid heartbeats, can reduce blood pressure and cause fainting. But they're much less dangerous than those involving the ventricles, the heart's lower chambers, which pump blood to the body. Since the treatment depends on the cause, your mother-in-law needs to be evaluated with a 24-hour Holter monitor, which should provide a diagnosis if the problem recurs while she's wearing it.

ASPIRIN FOR HEART ATTACKS

Q *If you think you're having a heart attack, is it better to chew an aspirin tablet or take a powdered aspirin product, like* BC Powder?

A Chew the aspirin tablet. *BC Powder* combines 845 milligrams of powdered aspirin (about 2.5 times the amount in a regular 325-mg adult aspirin) with 65 mg of caffeine, roughly the amount in a cup of instant coffee. That can be helpful for easing headaches, since caffeine can enhance the effects of pain relievers. But caffeine can also increase your heart rate and blood pressure, making the heart work harder, and it might cause extra heartbeats in people who are sensitive to it. And while powdered aspirin enters the bloodstream faster than a whole pill, chewing the aspirin has the same effect.

SURGERY FOR RACING HEART?

Q *Your article on atrial fibrillation didn't mention catheter ablation. Is that an effective treatment?*

A In many cases, yes. Atrial fibrillation is a rapid, irregular heartbeat caused by abnormal tissue in the heart muscle. The disorder can cause lightheadedness and fainting, and it increases the risk of heart failure and stroke. When medication fails to restore normal rhythms and there's no serious heart disease, a minimally invasive procedure called catheter ablation can be considered. During that procedure, a laser or radio-wave device is snaked through a vein up to the heart, where it destroys the abnormal tissue. That restores normal heartbeat in 70 to 90 percent of patients, though up to one-third may require additional procedures and up to one-fourth may still need drugs. About 1 to 2 percent of patients experience complications such as serious vein narrowing or blockage, transient ischemic attacks (tiny strokes), bleeding around the heart, or rhythm abnormalities requiring a pacemaker. Moreover, the long-term safety and effectiveness of catheter ablation are unknown.

ATYPICAL ANGINA?

Q *I've read that angina, the type of chest pain that signals coronary heart disease, is usually brought on by exercise and relieved by rest. I sometimes experience chest discomfort while resting but never while exercising. Could that discomfort still be angina?*

A It's unlikely. But an uncommon form of coronary disease can cause angina when you're resting or asleep—due to arterial spasm, not blockage. To rule out that possibility, your physician could have you wear a heart monitor for 24 hours. You should also have a treadmill exercise test, even though you haven't noticed the pain while exercising. If those tests find no sign of coronary disease, your physician will investigate other possible causes of your discomfort. It's most likely to be a temporary problem, such as heartburn or spasms of the esophagus. Occasionally, however, the discomfort reflects a chronic disorder, such as a hiatal hernia or gallbladder disease.

ACCURATE ANGIOGRAM

Q *Before I started a strenuous exercise program, my doctor ordered an exercise stress test to check my heart, even though I have no symptoms of coronary heart disease. That test was inconclusive, so I had a thallium stress test, which indicated some coronary disease. To confirm that finding, I underwent angiography, which found no sign of disease. Which test should I believe?*

A Angiography. That procedure, in which the coronary arteries are injected with dye and examined by X-ray, is the most accurate test for blocked coronary arteries. The two stress tests are safer and less expensive than angiography, which is why they're generally done first. However, it is possible for those stress tests to turn up positive when there's actually nothing wrong.

HEART PALPITATIONS

Q *I'm 62 and have had heart palpitations for years. What can you tell me about them?*

A "Palpitations" is a nonmedical term for any heart rhythm that feels abnormal. That can include extra beats, dropped beats, forceful beats, rapid beats, or irregular beats. For proper diagnosis the abnormality must first be "captured" on an electrocardiogram or on a 24-hour heartbeat recording. Palpitations can be caused by emotional stress, an overactive thyroid, certain medications, or diseases of the coronary arteries, heart muscle, or heart valves. Sometimes there's no detectable cause. At some point soon you probably should have your palpitations checked, but first try eliminating a few things on your own—caffeine (coffee, tea, cocoa, chocolate, soda), nasal decongestants, appetite suppressants—and see if it makes a difference.

A preventable cause of stroke

A 58-YEAR-OLD CLINICAL PSYCHOLOGIST, A LONGTIME FRIEND and patient, arrived at the emergency room one December evening two years ago having experienced sudden numbness and weakness in his right arm about an hour earlier. The symptoms disappeared in the ambulance on the way to the hospital and his physical exam was normal, but the ER doctor correctly decided to hospitalize him for observation for either a transient ischemic attack (TIA, a brief blockage of blood flow in the brain) or a stroke.

Imaging studies showed no evidence of a stroke or an obstruction to the flow of blood to the brain through the carotid arteries. His electrocardiogram and blood tests showed that no "silent" heart attack had occurred, and a 24-hour Holter monitor showed no abnormal heart rhythms, either of which might have predisposed him to a cerebral embolus, a clot that travels from the heart to the brain. He was discharged, on aspirin, after a day in the hospital, and came to see me later that week.

He confessed that he was so frightened by the episode that he didn't want to let the matter drop. He said he had experienced occasional prolonged episodes of shortness of breath over the past few months, not related to exercise. We agreed to use an ambulatory heart-rhythm monitor activated by a button pressed at the first sign of a symptom (in his case, shortness of breath). A week later, I had my answer. His breathless episodes were associated with atrial fibrillation.

Haphazard heartbeats

Of all the abnormal heart rhythms, atrial fibrillation is the most common. Normally, an electrical impulse from the right atrium, one of the heart's two upper chambers, activates the ventricles, the lower chambers, in a regular one-to-one sequence—60 to 80 regular impulses per minute from the atrium, 60 to 80 beats per minute in the ventricles. With atrial fibrillation, this orderly system goes haywire. Multiple sites in the left atrium fire haphazardly, as rapidly as 400 times per minute.

Fewer than half of those firings make it through to the ventricles, so the heart rate in atrial fibrillation is usually between 70 and 160 beats per minute, in a totally chaotic and irregular sequence. In some cases, the fibrillation goes on indefinitely, while other patients experience it only intermittently. Most people notice the abnormal heartbeat, but amazingly, a few, including the psychologist, don't feel it at all. In either case, the abnormal heartbeat decreases the output of blood, often resulting in shortness of breath, light-headedness, and fainting.

But the most devastating potential problem from atrial fibrillation is a stroke, which can result from the formation of clots in the blood that pools in the quivering atrium. Strokes are two to three times more common in patients with fibrillation than in those without.

Back in rhythm

The first treatment priority is to thin the blood to minimize the possibility of a stroke. Those with risk factors for a stroke—which include heart failure, hypertension, advancing age, diabetes, and a history of a stroke or TIA—should be on warfarin (*Coumadin* and generic). But this potent drug has drawbacks, such as the risk of bleeding complications and therefore the need for monthly blood tests. So people without stroke risk factors typically start on aspirin, which has fewer side effects.

Other priorities are to slow the heart rate and get the heartbeat back to a regular rhythm. Most people can't tolerate heart rates above 100 beats per minute. Beta-blockers, certain calcium-channel blockers, and sometimes digoxin (*Lanoxin* and generic) are used to slow the rate. Somewhat more controversial are procedures to restore normal rhythm. Most cardiologists make at least one attempt to shock the heart back to a regular rhythm. While such attempts are often initially successful, recurrences are common. Catheter ablation, performed by a specialty cardiologist called an electrophysiologist, is becoming more widely used. A catheter with a radio-frequency transmitter or a freezing tool is inserted into a groin vein and snaked up to the heart, where it zaps and destroys those errant electrical areas in the left atrium.

I referred the psychologist to a nearby medical center for a catheter ablation. The procedure was a success and now, totally without symptoms and his fears of having a stroke relieved, he is once again treating anxieties other than his own.

✚ *Office* Visit

Heart attack on a platter

A FEW YEARS AGO ON THANKSGIVING DAY I WAS CALLED TO the emergency room to see a 52-year-old high school football coach in the throes of a heart attack. In the whirlwind of activity to stabilize him before a transfer to a nearby medical center for angioplasty and stenting, I didn't have time to sit down with his wife to take a decent history until later that evening. "You couldn't possibly believe what he ate today," she said, and went on to describe a meal that could have fed his entire starting offensive backfield. He also had a high blood cholesterol level and a family history of early coronary disease.

In years gone by, skeptics wondered whether a single meal could actually trigger a heart attack. But over the past decade or two, we've learned a lot more about the physiological events that take place after eating a meal packed with carbohydrates, fat, and salt. Some research has found that it can set the stage for a heart attack, as happened to our football coach. For example, a study of 1,986 heart-attack patients presented at a meeting of the American Heart Association in 2000 suggested that an unusually large meal quadrupled the chance of having a heart attack within the next two hours.

The price of a pig-out

After a large meal (a Thanksgiving feast can easily exceed 4,000 calories), cardiac output of blood is increased and diverted to the intestinal circulation to aid digestion, which can take as long as 6 hours, leaving other organs, including the heart and brain, relatively deprived. The work involved in all this shunting around of blood might be the equivalent of vigorous sex or moderate exercise.

But that's not all. An increase in insulin, triggered by the carbohydrate content of the meal, can compound the situation by preventing normal relaxation of the coronary arteries. Triglyceride elevation, from the fats and carbs, can impair the function of the inner lining of the coronary arteries and cause those vessels to become less elastic and acutely inflamed. Increases in inflammatory markers such as C-reactive protein have been noted following a large, high-fat meal. And the rise in blood pressure that usually occurs after eating such a meal can cause those inflamed patches to rupture, which in turn can lead to blockages and heart attacks.

Gobbling down a huge dinner can have other health consequences, too. The prodigious amounts of gastric acid produced during the body's effort to digest the food can cause acid reflux that often goes on for many hours. The high fat content of a typical holiday feast can precipitate a gallbladder attack in people who have gallstones. The high salt content might trigger acute heart failure in someone with a history of that condition.

Add to those possibilities the sleepiness generated not only by the meal but also by the wine one might imbibe (making the drive home an accident waiting to happen), waking up the next morning with acute gout, plus the embarrassing flatulence, and you have many good reasons to revamp your eating habits at Aunt Fannie's fabulous feast this year.

The only thing you probably don't have to worry about is rupturing your stomach. That rarely happens because it can expand to accommodate nearly four times the normal volume of food.

Be a gourmand, not a glutton

So what's a formerly fearless foodie to do when gathered 'round the family dinner table groaning with potentially deadly goodies?

- Don't arrive famished. Have a snack an hour or two before.
- Stay away from the finger food at the hors d'oeuvres table.
- Eat the salad first.
- Use a salad plate instead of a dinner plate.
- Taste everything to your liking, but take small portions and resist seconds.
- Eat slowly, and participate in conversation.
- Skip the dessert, or at least go easy on it. Fruit is preferable.
- Limit alcohol intake to one glass of wine, and drink at least one full glass of water.

Cholesterol

GREAT CHOLESTEROL, CLOGGED ARTERIES

Q *My mother, who's in her 70s, has a great lipid profile: a low total-cholesterol level, a high level of the "good" HDL cholesterol, and low triglycerides. And she exercises every day. (On the down side, she is a bit nervous and has high blood pressure, which medication keeps under control.) Yet tests recently revealed partial blockage of a coronary artery. What else can she do to keep her heart healthy?*

A Partially blocked coronary arteries are not uncommon for a woman your mother's age. While blockage occurs most often in people with such risk factors as smoking, diabetes, obesity, physical inactivity, and unfavorable lipid levels, it can also occur in people without these conditions. There are some potentially helpful steps your mother could take.

Most important, all coronary patients should ask their doctor about taking daily low-dose aspirin to help prevent blood clots, which can trigger a heart attack. In addition, eating plenty of fruits, vegetables, and whole grains will supply lots of possibly heart-shielding antioxidants as well as B vitamins. (Such a diet may help fend off cancer as well.) Your mother should also consider taking a daily supplement containing 3 to 6 micrograms of vitamin B12 (which many people over age 50 cannot absorb adequately from food). And she may want to consider various relaxation techniques to reduce excessive stress, a likely coronary risk factor. Finally, if her "bad" LDL cholesterol is higher than 100 milligrams per deciliter—"great" for the normal population, but still too high for a coronary patient—she needs to lower her LDL further.

LOWER DOSAGE, FEWER SIDE EFFECTS?

Q *After taking 20 milligrams of pravastatin (Pravachol and generic) daily for a year, I have now brought my cholesterol level under control. I want to lower my dosage to 10 mg to minimize possible side effects, but my doctor says the higher dosage poses no additional risk. Is that true?*

A Yes. In theory, the lower the dosage of any medication, the lower the risk of side effects and the lower the cost. But with the change you're considering, any decrease in that risk would be minimal, particularly if you're not experiencing any side effects at your current dosage. And any possible benefit might be outweighed by a reduction in the medication's cholesterol-lowering effect. As for cost, the smaller dose would save you only a few cents per day.

FEED YOUR "GOOD" CHOLESTEROL?

Q *What foods should I eat to raise my "good" HDL but not my "bad" LDL cholesterol?*

A Individual foods can't do much for your HDL, which fights heart disease by dragging cholesterol out of the arteries. Only a few dietary items, notably alcoholic beverages and possibly grape juice, may increase HDL, and then only slightly. In contrast, regular aerobic exercise can boost HDL substantially.

But reducing your LDL, which dumps cholesterol into arteries, protects your heart more effectively—and there are several good ways to do that. Proven dietary steps include eating less saturated fat (mainly from animal foods), trans fat (from partially hydrogenated oils), and cholesterol (from eggs and meat) and getting more soluble fiber (from produce, legumes, and oats). Soy foods and possibly plant sterols (from margarine such as *Benecol*) may help, too. Nondietary steps include losing weight and building muscle.

DRUGS AND GRAPEFRUIT

Q *I take atorvastatin (Lipitor and generic) for high cholesterol and nifedipine (Procardia XL and generic) for angina every day. Is there any danger in eating grapefruit while taking those?*

A There could be. Several compounds in grapefruit can inactivate an intestinal enzyme that controls the absorption of statin drugs, such as atorvastatin, and calcium-channel blockers, such as nifedipine. That can cause potentially harmful increases of those drugs in the blood levels. So don't start consuming grapefruit or grapefruit juice while taking them. But if you've already been doing so, with good results and no signs of overdose, it may be wise to stick with the combination; abandoning the grapefruit could lead to reduced absorption and inadequate blood levels of the drug. Note that grapefruit can similarly interact with the anticonvulsant carbamazepine (*Tegretol* and generic), the antidepressant clomipramine (*Anafranil* and generic), and many other medications.

CONFUSION OVER HDL AND LDL

Q *You seem to discuss HDL and LDL as if they were two types of cholesterol. But then you say that both HDL and LDL transport cholesterol. I'm confused.*

A The terminology is confusing. HDL (high-density lipo-protein) and LDL (low-density lipoprotein) are not types of cholesterol. Rather, they're fat-protein compounds that transport cholesterol through the blood. (HDL tends to carry cholesterol away from the arteries, thus earning the title of "good" cholesterol;

LDL, or "bad" cholesterol, tends to deposit cholesterol in the walls of arteries.) Sometimes, though, HDL and LDL are used as shorthand terms to refer to the lipoproteins together with their cholesterol cargo.

STOPPING STATINS

Q *Once you start taking a statin drug to lower your cholesterol, can you ever stop?*

A Sometimes, if you're careful and work hard at it. Statins don't "cure" high LDL (bad) cholesterol; once you stop, it usually goes back up. But certain lifestyle changes might reduce or even eliminate your need for a statin, in two ways. First, switching to a diet that's low in saturated and trans fat and high in fiber can lower LDL. Second, whether you need a statin depends on not just your LDL but also your overall heart-attack risk. So if you lose excess weight, stop smoking, and lower your blood pressure, you might reduce your need for the drug. If you've made those changes and your LDL has dropped, talk with your doctor about lowering your dose and perhaps eventually eliminating the drug. But don't alter the dose without consulting him or her, and never stop abruptly. That could trigger a heart attack. For a comprehensive free report on the safety, efficacy, and cost of cholesterol-lowering statins, go to *www.crbestbuydrugs.org*.

JUMPING CHOLESTEROL

Q *According to a finger-prick test, my blood-cholesterol level was 197. Two months later, it was 272 on a fasting blood workup. My diet didn't change during that time. Is such a jump possible in only two months?*

A No. Cholesterol readings cannot vary that much, that soon. The finger-prick test was probably wrong. Squeezing the fingertip to draw blood produces secretions that dilute the blood and can lead to a falsely low reading.

EATING BEFORE CHOLESTEROL TESTS

Q *I had my cholesterol tested recently at a health fair. The previous day, I had eaten two meals with lots of fat and cholesterol. Did that throw off my cholesterol reading?*

A No. Levels of total cholesterol don't change that much from day to day. So you don't have to fast or worry about what you eat the day before a test. But if you were having blood drawn for a complete lipid analysis, including HDL cholesterol and triglycerides, then a 12- to 14-hour fast would likely be required.

ARE TRIGLYCERIDES A THREAT?

Q *What are triglycerides, and can they really harm my health?*

A They're an abundant type of fat in the bloodstream. Excess amounts can increase the risk of heart attack and stroke directly, by helping to clog the arteries and promoting blood clots. They can also increase risk indirectly, in two ways. The liver converts excess triglycerides into the "bad," artery-clogging LDL cholesterol. And triglycerides tend to displace the "good," artery-clearing HDL cholesterol from the proteins that haul fats through the blood.

So people should try to keep their triglyceride level below 150 milligrams per deciliter (mg/dl). Steps that can lower triglycerides include losing excess weight; cutting back on saturated fat, sugar, other carbohydrates, and dietary cholesterol; minimizing alcohol intake; exercising regularly; stopping smoking; and keeping diabetes well controlled. Fish oil supplements and prescription drugs such as fenofibrate (*Tricor*) and gemfibrozil (*Lopid* and generic) are sometimes necessary to lower very high triglyceride levels (over 400 mg/dl), which can harm the pancreas.

CHOLESTEROL AND COFFEE . . .

Q *I've read that unfiltered brewed coffee can raise blood-cholesterol levels. But what about instant coffee?*

A Apparently not. That's because the manufacturing process removes nearly all of the two compounds—cafestol and kahweol—responsible for the increased cholesterol levels.

. . . AND DECAF

Q *Does decaffeinated coffee contain the compounds that can raise cholesterol levels?*

A That depends solely on how it's prepared. The decaffeination process itself has no effect on the offending substances—cafestol and kahweol. But like regular coffee, decaf that's instant or drip-filtered will have virtually none of those chemicals.

Colon and rectal complaints

HEMORRHOID RELIEF

Q *I've suffered from hemorrhoids for years, and recently some of them may have prolapsed. Can drugs cure them, or should I consider surgery?*

A Unfortunately, no drugs can cure hemorrhoids, those sometimes painful clumps of blood vessels that erupt from the lining of the rectum. The problem worsens when the clumps prolapse, or protrude outside the anus. But you probably won't need surgery, which requires hospitalization and costs several thousand dollars. That's typically reserved for problems such as pain, incontinence, bleeding, or ulceration.

First, try the following simple and usually effective remedies: Consuming more fiber and water, and taking a stool-softening drug such as docusate (*Colace, Surfak,* and generic) can help prevent worsening. To ease the irritation, sit in a warm bath, use a general-purpose wet wipe, and apply a water-based (nonpetroleum) ointment such as *K-Y Jelly*. (Those products are just as effective as the special hemorrhoid ointments and wipes sold in drugstores.) For temporary relief, take acetaminophen (*Tylenol* and generic)--not aspirin or ibuprofen (*Advil* and generic), which can promote bleeding. And try to gently push the prolapsed hemorrhoids back into the rectum after each bowel movement.

If those steps fail, discuss nonsurgical removal with your doctor; it's an office procedure costing a few hundred dollars. The most effective procedure uses special rubber bands that cut off blood flow to the hemorrhoids, which fall off in a week or so. Other techniques destroy the clumps with infrared or radio waves.

INFREQUENT BOWEL MOVEMENTS

Q *I'm a 58-year-old man who has a bowel movement only once every three days or so. Could that be hurting my health?*

A Possibly, though the evidence is mixed. Researchers have long theorized that infrequent bowel movements could increase the risk of colon cancer by prolonging contact between the feces and the colon lining. At least two large population studies seem to support that theory: One found that people who didn't move their bowels daily had a one-third higher risk of colon cancer; the other linked fewer than three movements a week with more than double the risk. But two other studies, including the largest and longest one, which followed some 85,000 women for 12 years, found little or no connection.

Whether or not infrequent bowel movements increase the chance of colon cancer, they might be a symptom of that disease as well as of ovarian cancer and Parkinson's disease. So tell your physician about any change in your bowel habits that doesn't resolve itself within several weeks. To stimulate bowel movements, exercise regularly and consume lots of fiber.

DIET AND DIVERTICULOSIS

Q *Like many people my age (over 50), I have diverticulosis. My doctor has told me not to eat seeds and nuts and to avoid constipation. But I know people with the same problem who have been told to eat, avoid, or do different things. Could you provide some insight into this problem?*

A Diverticulosis is a common condition in which the inner lining of the intestine protrudes into the intestinal wall, forming small pouches in the wall of the colon. It affects one in four people by the age of 50 and is nearly universal by the age of 80. It's believed that our modern low-fiber diet is at least partly to blame.

Diverticulosis usually doesn't cause any symptoms, but some people with the condition do experience bloating, cramps, and changed bowel habits, such as constipation, diarrhea, or alternating attacks of both. Abdominal pain (especially low on the left side) accompanied by fever might signal the development of diverticulitis, an infection of the pouches. That can lead to abscess formation and to perforation of the bowel, which can cause peritonitis, a generalized infection of the abdominal lining.

To avoid those problems, switch gradually to a higher-fiber diet with more whole grains, fruits, and vegetables.

ANAL ITCHING

Q *I have been suffering from severe pruritus ani for nearly a year. To find relief from the itching, I've been to a family physician, a proctologist, four dermatologists, and an allergist. So far, no treatment has helped. Do you know of anything that might relieve my discomfort?*

A Since you've already seen seven doctors, they've probably ruled out the most common causes of anal itching: worms, hemorrhoids, fungal infections, skin fissures, sweating, irritants in food, and poor anal hygiene.

One possibility that's sometimes overlooked is neurodermatitis. This is not an actual nerve disorder but rather a lengthy cycle of itching and repeated scratching. It leads to gradual thickening of the skin around the anus, which then itches more than ever.

If neurodermatitis is indeed the cause of your condition, it may gradually abate if you force yourself not to scratch the thickened skin. When you're at home, applying an ice-cold compress to the irritated area can ease the urge to scratch. Since many sufferers scratch when they're asleep, you should keep your fingernails short and even wear soft mittens to bed. A hypnotist or psychotherapist might help you stop scratching.

BLOOD IN THE STOOL

Q *Microscopic traces of blood have been detected in my stool. Sigmoidoscopy revealed internal hemorrhoids near the entrance of the anus. Does this mean surgery, even though I've had no discomfort?*

A Not necessarily. Stool softeners *(Colace, Surfak,* and generic) or psyllium laxatives *(Metamucil, Mylanta Natural Fiber,* and generic) can reduce straining during bowel movements and may help stop the bleeding, just as they help prevent anal fissures. Antihemorrhoidal creams and suppositories are not particularly helpful for this problem. Like persistent fissures, persistent bleeding may require surgery. A colonoscopy should be done to rule out bleeding sources beyond the reach of a sigmoidoscope.

COLON CLEANSERS

Q *I regularly drink a laxative tea to cleanse my colon. Could that be harmful?*

A Yes, and there's no evidence that it has any benefits. Proponents of colon cleansing, or "detoxifying," claim that the practice removes built-up toxins, rejuvenates the digestive tract, and can even fight cancer. But there's no credible research to back up those claims. What's more, a healthy body doesn't need outside help clearing out toxins, nor does your digestive tract require restorative rest. Worse, the chronic use of laxatives can be dangerous, leading to fluid loss, dehydration, and electrolyte imbalances. To maintain colon health, eat a diet rich in fruits and vegetables and get regular exercise, which in addition to its many other benefits seems to help keep the colon working properly.

Cysts, lumps, and tumors

BENIGN BUMP OR PERILOUS GROWTH?

Q *I have a small, hard, brown bump on my leg. My doctor says it should probably be removed. But my dermatologist says it's a harmless dermatofibroma. Should I be worried?*

A Not if it's really a dermatofibroma. Those knots of benign fibrous tissue commonly appear on the legs where the skin has been mildly inflamed, by an insect bite or splinter, for example. Though often confused with moles, those nodules are harder, may itch, and are sometimes purple or red. And unlike potentially cancerous skin growths, they don't change shape or color, are uniformly colored, have clearly defined edges, and generally don't bleed. Removal is not only unnecessary but can also leave a scar larger than the original bump.

BODY BUMPS

Q *I have several egg-shaped growths on my body. Please explain whether these bumps, diagnosed as lipomas, are dangerous and how the condition can be treated. I would have quite a few scars if the lumps were all surgically removed.*

A Lipomas are benign, fatty tumors that are fairly common, typically appearing on the trunk, neck, and forearms. Usually they cause no discomfort and are best left alone. If you prefer to have them removed for cosmetic reasons, you can choose either conventional surgery or liposuction, in which a small tube inserted under the skin sucks out the fatty tissue, resulting in less scar formation. The rare lipoma that enlarges rapidly may harbor a cancerous growth, known as a liposarcoma, and should be removed surgically.

BENIGN CHANGES IN THE BREAST

Q *Six months ago I had a breast biopsy that showed benign changes—fibrocystic disease and intraductal hyperplasia. Is either of these linked to an increased risk of breast cancer in the absence of a family history?*

A Your risk of breast cancer is no greater than average. The conditions you mention are natural changes that occur over time. Fibrocystic "disease," a term that implies an abnormality or disorder, is a misnomer, since about half of all premenopausal women have it. It's really a catchall term for painful, lumpy breasts. Such lumps were once thought to be associated with increased cancer risk, but several studies have since dispelled that notion. Intraductal hyperplasia is a benign overgrowth of cells in the breast ducts, the tubes that carry milk to the nipple. Only when those cells start to appear abnormal on a biopsy does the risk of cancer increase. Symptoms of fibrocystic breast disease typically improve after menopause.

Dental care

HELP FOR TAINTED BREATH

Q *I have bad breath, even though I don't smoke and I carefully brush my teeth and floss. Could the odor stem from some problem inside my body?*

A Probably not, unless you have other symptoms as well. But first check whether you really do have bad breath by asking an unbiased source, such as your doctor. Research suggests that one in four people who think they have bad breath actually suffers from "halitosis phobia." If your breath consultant confirms the problem, try gently cleaning your tongue. Even with scrupulous brushing and flossing, some people accumulate odor-causing bacterial plaque on the back of their tongue, which can cause bad breath. To remove the plaque and odor from your tongue, use a regular toothbrush or a tongue scraper or toothbrush with an attached tongue-cleaning pad, sold at drugstores, usually for a few dollars. Studies have disproven the popular belief that digestive disorders can taint your breath. But in about 10 percent of cases, bad breath stems from problems that don't involve oral hygiene. Those include infection or even cancer of the ear, nose, sinuses, mouth, throat, or lungs; or diseases of the liver or kidneys.

CALCIUM FOR ORAL HEALTH?

Q *I'm a 42-year-old woman with receding gums and bone loss around my teeth. My dentist recommends that I take calcium supplements to delay further bone loss. Is this the best treatment for my condition?*

A There's no evidence that getting extra calcium will help reduce periodontal disease, which is what causes such bone loss. You should be evaluated by a periodontist. Treatment options range from periodic root planing to various surgical therapies.

ANNUAL X-RAYS

Q *I'm an adult with healthy gums who hasn't had a cavity in years. Do I really need the annual X-rays that my dentist recommends?*

A Probably not, if you don't have a history of cavities or diseased or receding gums. Instead, ask your dentist about having bitewing X-rays. They target specific teeth your dentist may be concerned about, every two or three years. A set of full mouth X-rays is generally necessary only every ten years. If you've changed dentists, be sure to have any previous X-rays forwarded, since your new dentist may want them to assess your dental health or track changes over time.

GENTLE GUM CARE

Q *My dentist recently recommended that I use a* Water Pik *oral irrigator. Since I've used it at near-maximum pressure, my gums have stopped bleeding. But your recent report on tooth care stressed the importance of gentle cleaning. Does that apply to my new device as well?*

A Yes. Intense water pressure can force bacteria through the thin walls of the gums, especially if you have a periodontal pocket, or space between the gums and teeth. (Pockets are often present if the gums have been bleeding a lot.) Such spread of bacteria can lead to a more serious condition, such as severe inflammation or even an infection that spreads beyond the gums. So if you're using an oral irrigator regularly, don't set it at more than half power—which should still be enough to improve your oral health. And remember, water treatment doesn't take the place of daily brushing and flossing, which are still the most effective self-care steps for keeping your gums and teeth clean enough to help ward off gum disease and tooth decay.

SPECIAL TOOTHPASTE FOR TENDER TEETH?

Q *Some of my teeth hurt when I brush, even though I have no cavities or gum disease. I'm considering one of those special toothpastes for sensitive teeth. Do they really work?*

A Yes. Such pain usually stems from gum recession, which exposes the sensitive roots. The special pastes contain chemicals that can block that pain. Since brushing too hard can increase gum loss and sensitivity, use a soft-bristle brush and a gentle touch. And avoid whitening or stain-removing toothpastes, which can be more abrasive. If those steps don't help after a few weeks, your dentist may treat the problem teeth with a fluoride gel, a varnish, or a bonding agent.

TOOTHBRUSH HYGIENE

Q *Can you reinfect yourself by using the same toothbrush after you've been sick?*

A Possibly, so it's best to throw it out once you're well. Your toothbrush collects germs from any environment where it spends time, including the place where you store it and, of course, your mouth. In theory, using the same toothbrush you used when you had a bacterial infection (like strep throat) or viral infection (like a cold or the flu) could re-expose you to the germs. While boiling your toothbrush might help kill them, it's also likely to damage the bristles. So it's better to start fresh. To minimize germs, rinse your toothbrush before and after use; don't store it in a covered container, which promotes bacterial growth; and avoid sharing toothbrushes. If you share a bathroom with someone, store toothbrushes so they don't touch.

✚ Office Visit

Is that dental X-ray necessary?

WITH JAY W. FRIEDMAN, D.D.S., M.P.H.

MANY YEARS AGO I REFERRED A WOMAN TO A RENOWNED periodontist. She told me a few years later that every year the good doctor exposed her to a full-mouth periapical X-ray that showed her teeth from root to crown. I told her that gum disease progresses very slowly and that she didn't need those yearly X-rays, which involve more than a dozen separate shots. She told her periodontist, and he told her to find another one— which was really good advice.

Used appropriately, dental radiography is a valuable tool that enables us to diagnose dental caries (cavities) that attack teeth; gum disease that destroys the bone around teeth; the position of unerupted wisdom teeth; the type and degree of orthodontic malocclusion; and many other conditions. But when overused, X-rays can expose patients to unnecessary radiation and expense in exchange for little or no benefit. Economics also factor in overuse: Dental X-rays are a large source of income for many practitioners. And some dentists think X-rays are necessary to protect them from malpractice suits, when in truth the best protection is proper dental practice.

X-rays you don't need

There are few evidence-based studies about the appropriate use of dental X-rays, but there's broad agreement that they shouldn't be overused because of the cumulative radiation risk, especially for children. One study, "Dental X-Rays and Risk of Meningioma," published online in the April 2012 issue of the *Journal of Cancer*, found an association between higher exposure to dental X-rays, especially during childhood, and the development of meningioma, the most common—and fortunately, usually benign—type of brain tumor.

No responsible dentist today would recommend annual full-mouth periapical X-rays like my patient had. But other types of X-rays are also used inappropriately. They include:

• Routine bitewings—images that show the crowns of upper and lower teeth—during annual checkups.

• Full-head and jaw X-rays (cephalographs) before starting routine orthodontic treatment.

• Panographs—panoramic images of the teeth and entire jaw—to evaluate temporomandibular joint (TMJ) pain.

• 3-D cone-beam computed tomography (the latest fad)—similar to a CT scan but with far more radiation exposure—for orthodontics or routine wisdom-teeth extractions.

We dentists are not infallible. It's easy for us to overlook a cavity, an abscess, or even a large cyst, all of which often take years to develop. That's why at each examination your dentist should look at previous X-rays as if they were brand new to make sure nothing was missed before deciding on whether additional ones are needed.

X-rays you do need

Here's my guide to the appropriate use of dental X-rays, which is consistent with the American Dental Association's guidelines.

Bear in mind that there are always exceptions to guidelines, but they should be based on symptoms that lead your dentist to suspect something is wrong.

Children. If there are no spaces between the teeth, bitewing X-rays of the rear teeth should be taken at the initial examination. Bitewings should be repeated in 18 to 24 months for children at low risk with few or no cavities, and in 12 to 18 months for children with many cavities.

Adults. Full-mouth X-rays (periapicals or a panograph) and bilateral bitewing X-rays should be taken at the initial examination. Copies of X-rays taken by a previous practitioner within the last few years can be used if the patient has no new symptoms. For adults with few or no cavities, repeat bitewings in two to three years. For cavity-prone adults, bitewings should be repeated in 18 months, which is about how long it takes for a new cavity to become visible on an X-ray. It's not necessary to repeat full-mouth X-rays in less than 10 years, if at all, in the absence of reasons to expect some new dental disorder.

For routine orthodontic treatment, wisdom-teeth extractions, and temporomandibular joint (TMJ/TMD) disorders, avoid full-head films, 3-D cone-beam computed tomography scans, and special TMJ X-rays.

Today's dentists are more open to consumer concerns but may still be resistant to change. You may have to be persistent in rejecting unnecessary X-rays.

Diabetes

ASPIRIN AND DIABETICS

Q *Is it true that aspirin can lower blood-sugar levels in diabetics?*

A Yes, but only with prolonged use and in large amounts (eight or more 325-milligram tablets a day). That reduction in blood-sugar levels can magnify the sugar-lowering effects of insulin and oral antidiabetic drugs. While such use of aspirin is generally safe for people with diabetes, they must be monitored closely by a physician.

DROWSINESS AFTER EATING

Q *I get extremely tired after eating. Could that signal something dangerous?*

A Probably not. It's more likely that the drowsiness comes from eating foods or meals that are high in calories, high in simple carbohydrates such as sugar, or both. Ingesting a lot of calories causes the body to slow down multiple systems, including the brain, to divert extra blood to the digestive system. The shift in resources can leave you feeling lethargic. And in some people, notably those with prediabetes, eating a large amount of sugar causes blood glucose levels to spike and subsequently crash, causing fatigue. In those cases, eating smaller and more frequent meals, limiting sugar intake, or both should help you feel more energized. If the changes don't help, you might ask your doctor whether a health issue might be the culprit—particularly diabetes, a food allergy, or a thyroid disorder.

✚ *Office* **Visit**

The other diabetes

A 43-YEAR-OLD KINDERGARTEN TEACHER WAS REFERRED TO ME after three months of frequent urination and a thirst so incessant that she constantly carried a bottle of water. This plus her recent weight loss would have made her a classic case of Type I diabetes mellitus, except for one catch: Her blood sugars were normal and there was no sugar in her urine, negating that diagnosis.

Instead, she turned out to have an uncommon—and easier to manage—disorder known as diabetes insipidus.

What's in a name?
Whereas the most common diabetes mellitus stems from an abnormality in the pancreas, kidney malfunction is the immediate culprit in diabetes insipidus. When operating normally, our two kidneys filter four ounces of blood every minute, remove the toxins and return about 99 percent of the cleansed fluid back to the body. What's left is excreted as urine. This important process is called concentrating the urine. When it fails, the body pours out large quantities of dilute urine and rapidly dehydrates if you don't drink copious amounts of fluid.

Diabetes mellitus also results in frequent urination, caused by the high glucose content of the urine. In the days before lab tests, doctors had to taste the urine to tell the difference between the two disorders. The sugar-laden urine of diabetes mellitus is sweet ("mellitus" being a Latin term for sweetened), whereas the dilute urine of the other diabetes is tasteless, or insipid.

What's at fault?
The ability of kidneys to concentrate urine depends on a

substance aptly called antidiuretic hormone (ADH). Made in the brain and stored in the pituitary gland, ADH is sensitive to hydration changes. If we drink too much, its release is inhibited so that we can easily excrete the added fluid and not get overhydrated. When we don't drink enough fluids, ADH is released and prompts the kidneys to reabsorb more water so we don't get dehydrated. Any glitch in this system will cause the kidneys to lose their urine-concentrating ability.

One rare cause is an inherited condition called nephrogenic diabetes insipidus, which may not become apparent until adulthood. Drugs that can impair the kidneys' ability to respond to ADH include lithium (most commonly used to treat manic-depressive illness), amphotericin B (for severe fungal infections), demeclocycline (an antibiotic), and methoxyflurane (an anesthetic gas). Any disorder or medication that causes a prolonged hike in blood calcium levels or low potassium blood levels can also paralyze the kidneys' ability to reabsorb water.

But the problem is usually at the other end of the system: a defect in the brain's ability to produce proper quantities of ADH.

Reaching a diagnosis

The method used in the diagnosis of diabetes insipidus, the water deprivation test, has not changed for decades. It's uncomfortable, but doesn't take long and usually provides the answer. I hospitalized our schoolteacher for the day and, as the test's name suggested, prohibited her from drinking so much as a drop of water. I even disconnected the faucets in her room's sink so she wouldn't be tempted to cheat. We took hourly urine specimens that were tested for concentration and weighed her to measure urine loss. In five hours she lost nearly five pounds of fluid and also failed to concentrate her urine, thus securing the diagnosis. I then gave her an injection of synthetic ADH to see whether her kidneys responded normally. They did, which ruled out nephrogenic diabetes insipidus as the cause of her symptoms.

On direct questioning, her husband eventually recalled that she had struck her head on the car door about two weeks prior to the onset of her symptoms, a mishap that she thought nothing of at the time. An MRI of her brain showed no abnormality that could have explained her symptoms. But that seemingly slight blow to her head presumably caused damage to the area in her brain responsible for ADH production. The damage is likely to be permanent.

I started her on twice-daily doses of ADH administered by nasal spray. Her urine output fell to normal, her thirst abated, and she returned to her normal lifestyle, freed from the worry of having to know the location of every accessible bathroom in town.

Diet and nutrition

SODIUM IN CHICKEN

Q *My husband is on a low-salt diet, so I was alarmed to learn that many cuts of uncooked poultry contain added sodium. How can I identify those cuts?*

A Check the labels. They must declare anything that has been added to the meat, such as "a solution of water, salt, and sodium phosphate" injected to help keep the food moist, tender, and tasty during cooking. Meats prepackaged in a processing plant will also carry a separate, nutrition-facts label listing the total amount of sodium per serving. (That label isn't required on meat packaged at the store.) The amount of injected sodium varies widely: We found chicken breasts with as little as 119 milligrams (mg) of added sodium per 3-ounce serving, and turkey breasts with as much as 373 mg, in addition to 40 to 50 mg of naturally occurring sodium. Those servings supply roughly 7 and 17 percent, respectively, of the recommended daily maximum, and that's for people who don't need to restrict their sodium intake.

FRYING WITH HEALTHFUL FATS

Q *Eating foods fried in oils that are high in saturated or trans fats is bad for your arteries. But is frying in unsaturated fats such as corn, canola, and olive oil a healthy alternative?*

A It's healthier—but hardly healthy. Unsaturated fats do tend to improve cholesterol levels, and saturated and trans fats do the opposite. But frying can undermine that benefit. For one thing, the grease gives any fried food far more calories than the same food cooked in other ways. Moreover, the high frying temperatures can destroy the vitamins, antioxidants, and other disease-fighting compounds in both the food and the oil. And the heat creates other substances that help cholesterol stick to artery walls. (Preliminary evidence suggests that oils high in polyunsaturated fats, such as corn, safflower, and sunflower, may generate more of those artery-clogging substances than predominantly monounsaturated oils, such as canola, olive, and peanut.) In addition, heating any oil repeatedly or lengthily may create potentially cancer-causing compounds.

BOTTLED WATER VS. TAP

Q *Is the water sold at stores safer than the water at home?*

A That depends on your local water supply. There's no conclusive evidence that either type of water is purer than the other in general. But bottled may be a better bet if your tap water contains excessive levels of any contaminants. Check the Consumer Confidence Report, which your local water supplier must mail to homeowners each July; tenants should be able to get it at their library. The report lists the average (and acceptable) levels of various contaminants in your local water—though individual homes may have higher lead levels, for example, because of soldered pipes. If you want more testing, information on state-certified drinking water laboratories is available from the EPA state certification officer in your area. The contact information for each state is available at *http://water.epa.gov/ scitech/drinkingwater/labcert/index.cfm*, or you can call your state health department. Using a water filter is usually cheaper than switching to bottled water. In general, the filter's instructions should reliably indicate which contaminants it can remove. If you opt for bottled water, choose a fluoridated type.

SMOKING OUT THE OMEGA-3s

Q *I know that fish is a rich source of heart-healthy omega-3 fatty acids. Does smoking or pickling reduce the omega-3s?*

A Yes, and it may pose health risks as well. For example, fresh salmon is high in omega-3s, but smoking reduces the amount by about 75 percent. Fresh herring is also high in those beneficial fats, but pickling apparently destroys about 30 percent of them. While that still makes pickled herring a relatively rich source of omega-3s, both pickling and smoking can deposit carcinogenic compounds on the treated food. Indeed, eating pickled or smoked foods several times a week or more has been linked to an increased risk of developing certain cancers. So while the occasional smoked or pickled snack shouldn't jeopardize your health, it's best not to eat them regularly.

TO PEEL OR NOT TO PEEL

Q *Does eating fruit and vegetable skins provide nutritional benefits?*

A Yes, but there may be hazards, too. Skins tend to be fairly high in insoluble fiber, which can lower the risk of some digestive disorders, and they're loaded with phytonutrients, which may help prevent many diseases. But conventionally grown produce is usually coated with tiny amounts of pesticide residues. With certain items—apples, bell peppers, cucumbers, eggplants, peaches, pears, sweet potatoes, and tomatoes—the pesticides may be trapped under a layer of wax. Whether it's harmful to consume those residues is not clear. For maximum safety, particularly with children, you could scrub produce in a highly diluted solution of liquid dish detergent, which should remove most of the pesticides and wax. Or you could peel it––especially apples, peaches, and pears, which may be waxed and have particularly heavy residues. Alternatively, choose organically grown produce, which harbors very little or no residue. Organic produce should still be washed to remove other contaminants.

ARE BANANAS BENEFICIAL?

Q *Your recent story on phytochemicals in produce didn't mention bananas. Don't they contain any of those potentially disease-fighting compounds?*

A Yes, but less than the average amount in other fruits and vegetables. That's mainly because the major phytochemicals tend to be the same pigmented substances that give produce its color. Brightly colored foods such as blueberries and kale are loaded with phytochemicals—but bananas are not, because their flesh is relatively pale. However, bananas contain plenty of other worthwhile nutrients, notably vitamin B6, vitamin C, and potassium.

THE POWER OF PULP

Q *I prefer to use a juicer and drink my vegetables. But I've heard that I'm throwing out nutrients with the pulp. Would it be healthier to blend some veggies and tomato juice together, and drink the slush, pulp and all?*

A Yes, though you might want to choose low-sodium tomato juice. Using a juicer is an easy way to reap most of the vitamins, minerals, and certain other disease-fighting substances from vegetables and fruits. But juicing strains out most of the fiber, and some of the vitamins and minerals. In contrast, using a blender retains everything in the produce. Drinking slushed fruits or vegetables can be even healthier than eating them whole, since you're apt to consume more of them.

DOES EGGPLANT PARMESAN COUNT?

Q *I love eggplant parmesan. But does it actually count as a serving of vegetables?*

A Yes—though it's not particularly healthful. The eggplant is usually salted, battered, and fried first, then topped with lots of tomato sauce and cheese. So a typical one-cup portion contains about 50 percent of your daily quota of artery-clogging saturated fat and 30 percent of your sodium. The eggplant itself contains only negligible amounts of vitamins, minerals, and fiber. Though the skin contains phytochemicals, or potentially disease-fighting substances, it's usually peeled off and discarded. The tomato sauce and cheese fortify the dish somewhat: The sauce is a good source of vitamins A and C as well as the antioxidant lycopene, which has been linked with a reduction in prostate-cancer risk. And the cheese is rich in calcium and protein.

VEGGIES AND BLOOD CLOTS

Q *I take a daily aspirin to prevent blood clots. But I also enjoy eating collard greens, kale, and spinach, all rich in vitamin K, which promotes blood clotting. Do I need to skip these greens?*

A No. Leafy greens do contain ample amounts of clot-promoting vitamin K. So eating them could weaken the effects of certain anticlotting drugs such as warfarin (*Coumadin* and generic), but only if you suddenly started consuming huge amounts of them. In contrast, aspirin prevents clots in a totally different way that's not affected by vitamin K, so you can enjoy all the healthful greens you want.

BAKED VS. SWEET POTATOES

Q *You said that regular potatoes have a very high glycemic load. Are sweet potatoes a healthier alternative?*

A Yes—but that doesn't mean you need to abandon regular potatoes. High-glycemic foods contain lots of easily digested carbohydrates that can rapidly raise blood sugar; some evidence suggests that a high-glycemic diet may increase the risk of heart disease and diabetes. A regular potato's glycemic load is very high, while a sweet potato's is roughly average. Moreover, sweet potatoes are higher in fiber and most nutrients than regular potatoes. Still, the regular kind of potato can add variety to your diet, as well as more folate than a sweet potato and moderate amounts of several other nutrients. So an occasional baked potato can still be a good nutritional choice, especially if the rest of your diet contains relatively few high-glycemic foods, notably sugar and refined flour.

DIGESTING FIBER

Q In a recent issue you said fiber slows the digestion of food. But I thought fiber helped to protect against colon cancer by speeding up digestion. Which is true?

A Fiber does slow digestion; however, it fights colon cancer by hastening the elimination of waste products. Some of the fiber you consume dissolves into a gel that slows the absorption of nutrients from the stomach and small intestine. That helps keep blood-sugar levels from spiking, which may help lower cardiovascular risk in susceptible people. Fiber can also discourage overeating by making you feel fuller. In contrast, the colon, or large intestine, plays only a limited role in the digestion of food but a major role in excretion. Fiber entering the colon helps create soft, bulky stools that speed the excretion of potentially cancer-causing wastes.

TYPES OF FIBER

Q A recent issue provided an interesting and useful article on fiber. Could you expand on the respective roles and importance of soluble vs. insoluble fiber?

A Many foods contain both types of fiber: soluble fiber, which dissolves in water, and insoluble fiber, which does not. The two types of fiber behave very differently inside your digestive tract. Soluble fiber, plentiful in beans, oats, some vegetables, and most fruits and whole grains, takes on a gelatinous consistency that will make you feel fuller and less inclined to overeat; it also helps to lower insulin and cholesterol levels. Insoluble fiber, found in whole grains, beans, most vegetables, and some fruits, absorbs water, making stools softer and bulkier. In theory at least, that may reduce the risk of colon cancer by speeding potentially cancer-causing wastes through the colon and also reducing their concentrations.

ARE NONPOISONOUS MUSHROOMS HARMFUL?

Q *I've heard that grocery-store mushrooms contain potentially harmful substances. Is that true?*

A Yes, but the actual risks are vanishingly small. Mushrooms contain purines, which can aggravate gout, and agaritine, which causes kidney, liver, or stomach cancer in lab animals. But so many foods contain purines that it's impractical for gout sufferers to restrict their diet; instead, they're usually advised to take antigout drugs such as allopurinol *(Zyloprim)* or generic probenecid. And mushrooms contain only a trace of agaritine. While no studies have examined its effects on humans, researchers estimate that if 10,000 people ate a serving of raw mushrooms every day for 70 years, agaritine would cause only one case of cancer. Cooking lowers the agaritine content by about a third, further cutting that risk. Moreover, mushrooms are rich in chemicals that appear to fight breast cancer and, in theory, other cancers as well. And they're generally good sources of protein, B vitamins, and several minerals.

STALE PRODUCE

Q *Does the nutritional content of fruits and vegetables change after they're harvested?*

A The mineral content doesn't. But in most vegetables, the vitamins and phytochemicals—potentially disease-fighting substances—generally start breaking down after harvest. In fact, frozen vegetables can be more nutritious than "fresh" items that are no longer very fresh. In contrast, the vitamins and phytochemicals in foods that keep ripening after they're picked—including fruits as well as tomatoes, peppers, and avocados (which are technically fruits)—generally increase until they're fully ripe. And scientists have just learned that certain nutrients also increase in at least some fruits that don't ripen, such as berries and cherries, after the fruit has been harvested and refrigerated.

ARE RUNNY EGGS RISKY?

Q *I like poached eggs with yolks that aren't fully firm. Am I risking a salmonella infection?*

A Yes, but the risk is quite small. The Food and Drug Administration has estimated that only 1 in 20,000 eggs contain salmonella bacteria. You can kill any bacteria and eliminate the slim chance of infection by cooking eggs till both the whites and yolks are firm. If you want runny yolks with no risk, look for pasteurized eggs, which are flash-heated to destroy any bacteria.

Salmonella poisoning causes fever, stomach cramps, and diarrhea that generally last about a week, occasionally requiring hospitalization. People with impaired immunity, pregnant women, infants, and older people are at increased risk of severe complications. So while other people can decide for themselves whether the risk warrants giving up runny yolks or unpasteurized eggs, high-risk individuals should take those precautions.

NUTRITIOUS COOKING

Q *What are the best ways to cook vegetables so they retain the most nutrients?*

A In a few cases, heating actually increases the availability of certain nutrients, such as the antioxidants in carrots, spinach, and tomatoes. But in general, heat and water can strip produce of valuable substances such as vitamin A, vitamin C, the B vitamins, and some phytochemicals, or potentially disease-fighting compounds.

That's why it's best to avoid boiling, which leaches nutrients into water that is then discarded. Stewing also draws beneficial substances into the cooking liquid, but they remain part of the stew. Baking, roasting, grilling, and frying typically don't use water but often do use oils, which add fat and calories. And the foods are exposed to higher temperatures for a longer time.

For the healthiest results, use a microwave, steamer, or pressure cooker, which all preserve nutrients about equally well.

VEGETABLES VS. FRUITS

Q *You recently told a reader who ate lots of fruit to add some veggies, too. My question is the opposite: I eat lots of vegetables but little fruit. Am I missing out nutritionally?*

A Probably not much, though eating a variety of both vegetables and fruit is still the best approach. Fruits tend to provide more soluble fiber, which helps lower cholesterol levels, than vegetables do. But while both food groups are generally rich in vitamins and minerals, vegetables tend to supply more B vitamins, calcium, iron, and phytochemicals, or potentially disease-fighting plant compounds. And while numerous studies have linked a high intake of either fruits or vegetables with reduced risks of hypertension, coronary heart disease, and cancer, vegetables appear to provide more protection against certain cancers than fruits do. So while adding fruit might make a vegetable-rich diet even more nutritious, the vegetables alone should already be providing ample nutritional benefits.

COMPLETE PLANT PROTEINS

Q *I eat a lot of rice and beans, but I've heard that neither of them is a complete source of protein, since each is missing essential amino acids. How should I combine them to get enough complete protein?*

A Don't bother. If you're eating the recommended two to three servings of dairy plus a modest amount of meat each day, you're almost surely already getting enough protein. Even if you consume mainly plant proteins, trying to balance a few specific foods isn't necessary. Instead, eat a wide variety of legumes, nuts, seeds, grains, and vegetables throughout the day. That will supply your body with enough essential amino acids to manufacture the complete proteins that may be missing from individual items.

SMOKED MEAT AND CANCER

Q *Can eating smoked meat or fish increase the risk of cancer?*

A Possibly. A few studies have found that consuming those foods a couple of times a week or more increases the risk of developing certain cancers. That's because the smoke from burning wood contains large amounts of carcinogenic carbon compounds. Such compounds are found in many smoke flavorings as well as in smoked foods. Further, the preservatives used in many smoked products may react with compounds in meat to form additional carcinogens. So while the occasional smoked snack shouldn't jeopardize your health, frequent consumption of such foods should be avoided.

MICROWAVE COOKING

Q Does microwave cooking cause any loss of nutrients or other unhealthful change?

A Microwave cooking may actually retain nutrients better than traditional methods. That's because the longer you cook food, particularly in water that's discarded before eating, the more nutrients are lost. For example, one study found that spinach retained 100 percent of its folate—a water-soluble B vitamin—when cooked in a microwave, vs. 77 percent when stove-top boiled. Moreover, briefer cooking of meats produces lower levels of potentially cancer-causing chemicals.

But microwaving tends to heat foods unevenly, so the outer portions may not get hot enough. To help ensure germ-killing temperatures throughout, cover the food, leaving a hole for steam to escape. (Waxed paper is preferable to plastic wrap, which might transfer possibly harmful amounts of plastic to the food. For the same reason, use only containers labeled "microwave safe.") Stir and turn the food during cooking and let it stand for a while afterwards, as directed. And check its temperature in several places with a food thermometer.

EATING VEGETABLE LEAVES

Q *Are there benefits to eating the leaves (tops) of beets and other root vegetables?*

A It depends on the vegetable. Beet greens are high in potassium and vitamin A and can make a great side dish or addition to a salad. Note that they might begin to spoil before the beet root does. Turnip leaves are also healthful, with high levels of beta carotene, calcium, folate, and vitamin K. And both beet and turnip greens have plenty of fiber and disease-fighting phytochemicals. They're a better choice than carrot greens, which can contain alkaloids or other compounds that can cause illness, especially in sensitive or allergic people. It's best to skip them or limit their use to a garnish or minor salad ingredient. Avoid greens that are decayed or wilting, and wash them well before eating.

ONION EATERS

Q *Does eating onions provide me with any health benefits?*

A Green onions (such as scallions) have plenty of potassium and vitamins A and C. But most onions are very low in vitamins and minerals. However, like other "allium" vegetables—garlic, chives, leeks—all onions are rich in potentially disease-fighting substances, particularly sulfur compounds. Those compounds may help inhibit blood clots, reduce cholesterol levels, relax the arteries, and block the formation and effects of cancer-causing chemicals. Moreover, certain indigestible carbohydrates in onions, called oligosaccharides, may help speed the passage of cancer-causing substances through the colon. All those actions may help explain observational findings that link eating onions and other allium vegetables with reduced risks of colon and stomach cancer, lower cholesterol levels and blood pressure, and reduced risk of coronary heart disease. So in theory, eating onions and related vegetables may enhance your body's disease-fighting abilities.

A MORE NUTRITIOUS CHEESE?

Q *Are there any nutritional differences between soft and hard cheeses?*

A Ounce for ounce, hard cheeses tend to offer a better nutritional profile than soft cheeses. That's mainly because cheese loses moisture as it ages and hardens. So each serving of the harder types generally packs more calcium, protein, and minerals than the softer, younger types. Moreover, the harder, aged ones—excluding grating cheeses like Parmesan—tend to contain less sodium, because they're generally more flavorful, so less salt is needed to enhance their taste. There's no consistent connection between firmness and fat content. However, lower-fat versions of virtually any cheese typically provide 25 to 50 percent less fat than the regular versions and at least as much of the beneficial nutrients.

YAMS VS. SWEET POTATOES

Q *What's the difference between yams and sweet potatoes? And do all yams and sweet potatoes have "natural estrogen"?*

A In the U.S. some people use the word "yam" to describe the moister, sweeter, orange-fleshed variety of the familiar Thanksgiving root and reserve "sweet potato" for the drier, yellow-fleshed version. But most people use the terms interchangeably. Both varieties provide loads of carotenoids (many of which are precursors of vitamin A) plus a good supply of vitamin C, fiber, protein, calcium, magnesium, and potassium. However, neither variety bears any relation to "true" yams, which are much larger roots—generally at least 18 inches long, sometimes much larger—commonly eaten in Africa, Asia, and the Caribbean, but usually available here only in specialty markets. True yams are low in carotenoids but are otherwise just as nutritious as sweet potatoes. At least one type of true yam—the Mexican wild yam—contains chemicals that the body converts into the female hormones estrogen and progesterone. Limited research suggests that American yams and sweet potatoes probably have at most only a small amount of those chemicals. Mexican wild yam is used in some "natural estrogen" or "phytoestrogen" supplements.

BEST BITS OF BROCCOLI

Q *What is the most nutritious part of the broccoli plant?*

A The florets contain substantially more cancer-fighting phytochemicals and beta-carotene (a precursor of vitamin A) than the stalks, and about the same amounts of minerals and vitamin C. Whether you're eating the florets or the stalks, broccoli that's raw or lightly cooked (by microwaving or steaming) will supply the most nutrients. For a healthy sandwich or salad topping, look for broccoli sprouts, which pack 20 to 50 times more phytochemicals than the full-grown plant and comparable amounts of vitamins and minerals.

DRIED-FRUIT FACTS

Q How do dried fruits stack up nutritionally against fresh ones?

A Better in some ways, worse in others. Reducing the water content of fruit concentrates its fiber and minerals, certain vitamins (notably vitamin A), and many phytochemicals, potentially disease-fighting substances found in plants. But the sugar and calorie contents rise by comparable amounts. Moreover, drying destroys the water-soluble vitamins, including C and the B vitamins, as well as certain heat-sensitive phytochemicals. So while dried fruits can supply a lot of certain nutrients, a balanced daily diet should include at least some fresh fruits plus a few servings of vegetables. (Note that dried fruits treated with sulfites retain more of their color, vitamins, and phytochemicals than untreated fruits, but they can cause allergic reactions or asthma attacks in susceptible individuals.)

MUST EVERY MEAL BE BALANCED?

Q For several years, I've conscientiously tried to eat a healthy, balanced diet every day. Now I read that for best results, every meal must be balanced. Is that true?

A No. Your body has enough reserves of various nutrients to thrive for a while if some meals are unbalanced, or even missed. For example, foods that provide energy—protein, carbohydrates, and fats—should be replenished daily. Water-soluble vitamins, including the B-complex vitamins and vitamin C, will last two to three days. Your body stores enough minerals and fat-soluble vitamins, such as A, D, and E, to last weeks or even months.

DIGESTING SOYBEANS

Q *I can no longer eat beans because they give me gas and intestinal cramps. If I eat tofu, will I have the same problems?*

A Processed soy products such as tofu are less likely to cause intestinal discomfort. Soybeans and other legumes contain carbohydrates called oligosaccharides, which the body can't digest since it lacks the necessary enzyme, alpha-galactosidase. So the intact oligosaccharides move on to the lower intestine, where they're broken down by bacteria, producing gas. The processing of soy products such as tofu, tempeh, miso, and soy "protein isolate" removes the oligosaccharides; all of these products are easier to digest than whole soybeans. You can eliminate most oligosaccharides from raw beans by soaking them overnight. You might also try *Beano*, a product that provides the missing enzyme. (People with diabetes should check with their doctor before taking *Beano*, since the enzyme produces a type of sugar that might hinder their blood-sugar control.)

LEAFY GREENS AND BLOOD CLOTS

Q *I was recently prescribed warfarin* (Coumadin *and generic*) *for the prevention of blood clots. My doctor warned me to remove leafy green vegetables such as lettuce, brussels sprouts, cabbage, and broccoli from my diet. Is it really necessary for me to avoid such nutritious foods?*

A No. It's true that leafy green vegetables contain vitamin K, which tends to counteract the anticlotting actions of warfarin. So in theory, eating lots of leafy greens might make warfarin less effective—but only to a relatively small extent. And that effect shouldn't matter at all, since the warfarin dose should be adjusted regularly, based on your blood-clotting time while you're on your usual diet, including whatever amount of leafy greens you habitually eat. The only precaution you need to follow is that you shouldn't drastically change your intake of leafy greens—or any other part of your diet—while you're on warfarin, since that conceivably could alter your clotting time and, in turn, your need for the drug.

NUTRITIONAL INSURANCE

Q *I like to drink* Ensure *since I think my diet might be subpar. Is that a good idea?*

A Maybe. Liquid nutrition supplements such as *Ensure* and *Boost* can provide nourishment to people who are too ill or frail to consume adequate calories or who need extra nutrients because of a digestive disorder or a disease such as cancer. It's best to limit use of the drinks to those situations for a couple of reasons. An 8-ounce bottle contains about 350 calories—more than triple the amount in a can of soda—and about 20 grams of sugar. That's OK if you're struggling to get enough calories but not so good if you're overweight. And snacking on the drinks could crowd out healthier foods such as fruits, vegetables, and whole grains, which provide fiber and many other beneficial substances.

ARE SOY NUTS REALLY NUTS?

Q *A recent issue recommends nuts as a heart-healthy snack food. Does that suggestion include soy nuts as well?*

A Yes, we heartily recommend filling your nut dish with soy nuts. However, soy "nuts" are actually roasted soybeans—a type of legume. Like actual nuts, soy nuts are rich in nutrients, including protein, vitamin E, potassium, and fiber, that may help reduce the risk of coronary heart disease. At about 130 calories per 1-ounce serving, soy nuts contain roughly 25 percent fewer calories and significantly less total and saturated fat than an equivalent serving of peanuts (another legume) or real nuts such as almonds, cashews, and walnuts. Years ago, the Food and Drug Administration concluded that 25 grams a day of soy protein (found in soy nuts and other foods made with soybeans), combined with a diet low in saturated fat and cholesterol, may help reduce the risk of coronary heart disease by lowering blood-cholesterol levels. Soybean-based foods that meet certain FDA requirements can now include that health claim on their label. (A quarter-cup serving of soy nuts contains a little more than 8 grams of soy protein.)

OMEGA-3 SOURCES

Q Can I get omega-3 fatty acids from fresh-water as well as ocean fish?

A Yes. Lake trout is one of the richest sources of omega-3s, the healthful fatty acids that have been linked to a decreased risk of cardiovascular disease. In general, though, fish with high levels of omega-3s tend to be oily ocean-dwellers that live in cold water, such as salmon, herring, and pollock. Those species also tend to have lower levels of mercury, making them a safer choice than some other ocean fish. (Opt for wild, or Alaskan, salmon, which is usually lower in contaminants called PCBs than farm-raised salmon.) Most people can meet the recommended intake of omega-3s by eating two to three servings of fish a week. Those who don't like seafood can consider fish-oil pills. (Look for ones labeled "USP Verified.")

WHEN TO DRINK WATER

Q *I received a chain e-mail message that said it's more important to drink water at certain times of the day than at others. Any truth to that?*

A Probably not. It's true that your body needs ample water each day from food and beverages to maintain proper function. But there's no evidence that drinking it at specific times—say, first thing in the morning, to "activate your organs"—correlates with better health. If you don't drink enough fluids, it might be helpful to drink water at certain times, such as during meals, so you won't forget to do it. Otherwise, you can generally let thirst and activity guide you. You should drink some water before, during, and after vigorous exercise to prevent dehydration. You might also need to increase your intake in very hot weather. But avoid drinking excess fluids right before bed, which could interfere with another function: sleep.

SUGAR IN FRUIT

Q *Do some types of fruit have a lot more sugar than others?*

A Yes—but don't let a diet that demonizes carbohydrates convince you that it's bad to eat certain fruits. The sugar in fruit can range from 0 grams in an avocado (yes, it's a fruit) to 26 grams in a medium-sized pomegranate, with most fruits providing somewhere between 6 and 12 sugar grams per serving. While all sugar adds calories to your diet, there are a lot of good reasons to choose fruit over nutritionally empty sweets like candy or soda. It takes longer to digest and doesn't cause the spike in blood sugar (and subsequent hunger-inducing plummet) that the refined sugars in processed sweets do. Fruit is often packed with fiber and water, both of which can help you feel full. And it's a great source of disease-fighting vitamins, minerals, and phytochemicals. Moreover, giving healthful foods like fruit a prominent role in your diet leaves less room for the unhealthy stuff.

MIDNIGHT CRAVING

Q *Lately I have been waking up in the middle of the night craving, then devouring, sweets. What could cause that?*

A The problem is common enough that doctors have a name for it: night-eating syndrome. People who have it typically have little appetite in the morning but get very hungry at night. They overeat in the evenings, often have difficulty falling asleep, and wake up during the night to eat more. It appears most common among people who have depression or diabetes, or those who are severely obese. Psychotherapy, sometimes along with an antidepressant drug, may help reduce symptoms. Prescription sleep drugs such as zolpidem (*Ambien* and generic) can, in rare cases, cause "sleep eating," sometimes with no memory of it the next day. If that's the case, consider a different drug, or better yet, nondrug measures that can improve sleep.

GOOD GRAPES

Q *I've read about the benefits of resveratrol from wine. Can I get some of the same benefits from grape juice?*

A Probably. Red wine, grapes, and grape juice, as well as raspberries and peanuts, are all good sources of resveratrol, an antioxidant that's been shown in some animal studies to help prevent certain cancers, diabetes, and age-related decline in cardiovascular function. (It comes from the nonalcoholic component of wine.) Studies of resveratrol's effect on human cells have yielded some positive results, but it's not clear whether the benefits shown in animal studies will apply to humans, too.

SALT SUBSTITUTES

 I'm trying to cut back on salt. Is it worth trying a salt substitute?

Possibly, but not all of them are safe for everyone. Products like *No Salt Original* and *Nu-Salt* contain potassium chloride rather than sodium chloride. Potassium can help lower blood pressure and may reduce the risk of strokes and heartbeat abnormalities. But most Americans get plenty of the mineral from foods, including bananas, kiwis, milk, nuts, and yogurt. And extra potassium can be dangerous for people who have kidney disease or take certain drugs for heart disease, high blood pressure, or liver disease. They should talk with a doctor before using a salt substitute. Even when salt substitutes are safe, a 2008 Consumer Reports test found that those with potassium chloride have a bitter or metallic taste. So you might instead try to cut back on salt by adding herbs and spices to food.

RADIATION FROM BANANAS

I hear that bananas are radioactive. Should I be concerned about eating them?

No. Bananas naturally emit small amounts of radiation due to their high level of potassium, which is among a handful of elements that contribute to what's knows as "background radiation." That's the radiation that naturally exists in the environment, which we're continuously exposed to by way of food, water, and air. The radiation you get from a banana is so small it's inconsequential: about 0.00007 millisieverts, vs. 0.1 mSv from a chest X-ray and 10 mSv from a full-body scan. That tiny amount is extremely unlikely to have any bearing on cancer risk. And the benefits of eating bananas outweigh any potential risks, since they contain fiber and vitamin B6, as well as potassium, which helps regulate blood pressure and maintain muscle function.

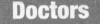

Doctors

WHAT DOES A D.O. DO?

Q *Can you tell me what the difference is between a D.O. and an M.D.?*

A D.O. (doctor of osteopathy) receives a medical education that's basically equivalent to that of an M.D. (doctor of medicine). Osteopaths are trained and licensed to perform all aspects of traditional medical care—including diagnosis, drug prescription, and surgery. In fact, they can specialize in virtually any area of medicine, although most choose primary care.

The difference between the two degrees is that osteopaths are also trained in osteopathic medicine, which emphasizes how the musculoskeletal system, particularly the spine, affects the entire body. They diagnose and treat certain conditions by manipulating joints. That can mean stretching the wrist of someone with carpal-tunnel syndrome or manipulating the spine to treat low-back pain, for example. Some osteopaths also use such therapy along with conventional treatments to ease the discomfort of conditions such as asthma, migraine, and pneumonia.

Office Visit

Your symptoms: Say what you mean

HIS PROBLEM WAS PERSISTENT DAILY HEADACHES THAT BEGAN THE previous winter as soon as the weather turned cold. At about that time, this 37-year-old systems analyst had taken a faster-paced, better-paying job that he hoped would enable him to buy a home and replace the 20-year-old jalopy he had to drive an hour each way to and from work. After a workup that included a referral to a neurologist, CT scans and MRIs of his head and neck, and a complete laboratory survey, his doctors decided the long commute and increased job stress were causing tension headaches. But *Valium* and several muscle relaxants didn't help. Some well-meaning friends suggested he get psychiatric help. He remained miserable.

When I questioned him closely, I learned that his headaches waned noticeably several hours after he arrived at work and returned soon after he got home in the evening, yet they never bothered him on weekends. Those details gave me a hunch. I asked him to drive straight to my office after work one evening. He arrived with a splitting headache. A blood test showed an elevated level of carboxy hemoglobin, an indicator of carbon-monoxide poisoning. He got rid of that car so fast that we never found out the source of the exhaust leak that nearly cost him his life. His headaches disappeared just as fast.

Communicate your condition

For many people the notion of modern medical diagnosis conjures up images of assorted high-tech tests, computer analyses, and complex imaging equipment. All these tools do help enormously in diagnosing disease, yet none is more important than the patient's ability to explain his or her case to the doctor. Inadequately expressed symptoms can lead even good physicians down the garden path to misdiagnosis. If you do your part by communicating your symptoms accurately and forcefully, your doctor stands the best chance of getting to the bottom of your problem. Here's how:

- **Get the timeline right.** Take along a written list of all of your complaints and do your best to list them in chronological order. Knowing which symptoms came first can often be the decisive factor in arriving at a workable diagnosis—as it was with the systems analyst's headaches.

- **Get down to business quickly.** Time-stressed doctors have a tendency to narrow down the list of possible diagnoses fairly quickly after an office visit begins. You need to make your concerns known at the outset before your physician jumps to what may turn out to be an erroneous conclusion.

- **Be specific.** Instead of complaining vaguely about pain, rate it on a scale of zero to 10 (with 10 being the worst). Describe the quality of the pain. Is it dull and aching, as with tooth pain? Does your chest feel on fire, as with heartburn? Does the pain sting like an insect bite? Or is it a painful pressure, as if an elephant were sitting on your chest? Does the pain radiate, or spread, into adjacent areas? How long has it hurt, and how often does it hurt? Do changes in your position, exercise, sexual activity, or emotional state affect the pain? Does anything make it feel better? Or worse?

- **If you fear the worst, say so.** If you dismiss abdominal pain as "probably just gas," your doctor may be tempted to agree—even if you're secretly worried about ovarian cancer. I once saw a patient who had undergone six months of psychiatric treatment for a presumed anxiety syndrome. Numerous tests seeking a physical cause for her lightheadedness, sweating, and shakiness had come up negative. Careful questioning revealed that her symptoms kicked in only when her heart skipped a beat or two. Once I reassured her that the occasional missed beats were normal, the symptoms disappeared.

- **Practice full disclosure.** Be sure to tell your physician about visits to other doctors or specialists. Different specialists, each scrutinizing seemingly unrelated symptoms, can miss the forest for the trees. A recent example is a 43-year-old woman who saw a cardiologist for her high blood pressure, an orthopedist for her backaches, an internist for her diabetes, and a neurologist for her headaches. It turned out that all those problems stemmed from a single cause—a pituitary tumor causing Cushing's disease, an uncommon disorder that in turn caused her adrenal glands to produce too much cortisol. That potentially fatal condition had gone undiagnosed—and untreated—for nearly five years because this patient had not discussed all her symptoms thoroughly with any one physician. When she finally got around to doing so, her combination of symptoms prompted appropriate testing—and an eventual cure.

✚ *Office* **Visit**

How to haggle with your doctor

WITH JOHN SANTA, M.D., M.P.H.

It's hard to listen to the news these days and not wonder whether you, like so many other Americans, could end up drowning in health-care bills. Sure, you're probably insured. But more and more folks with health insurance are facing large deductibles, plus paying an increasingly large portion of the rest of the bill. So it's important that you become a savvy health-care buyer—and even be able to haggle if you have to. Here's advice for three possible scenarios.

You're healthy. This is the optimal time to talk with your doctor about costs: before you've incurred any. Having a practitioner you trust is key. Physicians, nurses, and other providers have a professional obligation to take your financial resources into account when recommending and delivering care. But you might have to let them know that costs are important to you, especially since some practitioners are liable to suggest the most aggressive —and usually most expensive—options first. (The reasons for that are complicated, ranging from a patient's preferences to the fear of malpractice suits to pure financial motivation.)

Once you let your doctor know that cost matters, you might be surprised by the reasonable, more conservative options he or she comes up with, such as recommending a different drug regimen that involves fewer brand-name prescriptions or choosing watchful waiting over a costly diagnostic test that's not likely to affect the course of treatment. Having a good relationship with a doctor can also be helpful if you wind up in a dispute with a hospital or other health-care provider, since your doctor can go to bat for you to dispute the costs.

The unexpected occurs. You went into the hospital for a coronary angiogram and expected to pay a few thousand dollars: now you've been slammed with a $15,000 bill that's way beyond your resources—and your insurance is covering only a portion. If possible, sit down with the doctor who ordered the procedure and go over the bill together to see how the costs ran so high. Make sure all the hospital services were needed and reasonably priced; you can look up the going rate in your area for many medical services at *www.healthcarebluebook.com*, a free resource that provides information on health-care costs and advice to consumers. Examine hospital bills closely for errors, which are common.

Don't assume the price on your bill is set in stone. Providers often discount rates substantially to insurers and others, so why not ask whether you, too, might get a reduced rate? Dispute any charges you think your insurance company should cover, and don't pay until you have exhausted all your options. Do make clear to the hospital's billing department that you're willing to work toward a resolution, and consider making a discounted offer that you can manage within a set period. You can also consult one of the reputable groups that, for a fee, can help to reduce the size of medical bills, such as INSNET (*www.myinsnet.com*) or Medical Cost Advocate (*www.medicalcostadvocate.com*)

You're having an elective procedure. This situation is a bit less daunting, since you have some time to research the best device, doctor, hospital, drug, or other option, and should have the funds to cover the procedure. Do the research. Variations in health-care costs can be stunning, and plenty of providers will gladly let you overpay for a service that you could get for less.

As with any purchase, beware of shortcuts, too-good-to-be-true offers, and providers you've never heard of. Don't hesitate to ask for the price up front and get it in writing. Request an itemized list of all potential charges—not just, say, what the cosmetic surgeon will charge to do your eyelids but what you'll pay at the hospital or outpatient clinic where the procedure takes place (which often far exceeds the doctor's charges). Shop around, talk to providers, and bargain for what you think is a fair price.

✚ *Office* **Visit**

Six things to do in a doctor's waiting room

WITH ORLY AVITZUR, M.D.

WAITING FOR A DOCTOR CAN GET FRUSTRATING, ESPECIALLY IF you're in a hurry. Just last week I cooled my heels for more than an hour when I took my son to get a flu shot. While I paced, he texted his friends (and the doctor kept coming out to check the football game scores). As a physician myself, I got to thinking there must be things patients can do to make their wait more productive and less irritating. The next time you're kept waiting, you may want to consider these:

1 Make a list of your top health concerns

If you organize them in advance, it can help us concentrate on your problem and provide you with optimal treatment. If you're a new patient, we want to know the main reasons you're here. If you're a returning patient, we'd like to hear how you've been feeling since your last appointment. Focus on your most frequent or most severe symptoms, noting when they began, how often they occur, what makes them worse, and what makes them better. Try to keep your explanations clear and to the point, without too many tangents. That will help us evaluate your complaints and arrive at the right diagnosis. And bring complaints up early enough during your visit to discuss them. Nothing's more disruptive than a patient who mentions an urgent symptom just as we're about to move on to the next patient.

2 Write questions down

It's the easiest way to remember to ask them, and it will save you the hassle of making a follow-up phone call. Glance at the list as your appointment is winding down to see whether you've covered everything. It can also be useful to repeat the answers back to your doctor. That helps avoid potentially dangerous misunderstandings.

3 Make a list of all your medications

I've seen more medication errors than I care to admit. Some were due to drug interactions, others to dosage errors, and still others to drug-name mix-ups. That's why I advise all of my patients to keep a complete list in their wallet of all the prescriptions, over-the-counter drugs, and dietary supplements they take, and update it whenever there's a change. Ideally, this is something you should take care of well in advance of your appointment. One of my patients, for instance, writes her list on an index card cut in half, then covers it with clear, extra-wide packing tape. People who prefer computerized lists can use software programs like MedHelper, MedCoach, and others available online. That's how one of my favorite patients has been keeping me updated for the past 10 years, and he's 94! If you haven't planned ahead, though, now's a good time to get started.

4 Ask the office to check on your test results

We're better able to give you answers during your visit if we have all your test results on hand, something that can't be taken for granted in our fragmented system. If you've had any tests done since your last visit—laboratory work, scans, X-rays—ask the receptionist to see if the results are on file. If not, there may still be time to get the reports faxed to the office before your appointment starts.

5 Confirm that the office has the correct insurance information

We need this to get pre-authorizations for diagnostic tests and referrals to specialists, and to make sure that billing goes smoothly. Incorrect or expired information can hold up your treatment and lead to billing hassles later for you and your doctor.

6 Read something besides the magazines

In addition to brochures and pamphlets from patient organizations, waiting rooms often have reprints of articles we've found particularly helpful. While the Internet can be a great source of medical information, much of the material in our offices provides the added advantage of having been vetted. Just make sure you check the source; pharmaceutical company sales representatives like to leave promotional material, and they don't always ask for permission.

Ear problems

TUNING OUT TINNITUS

Q Is there any cure for chronic ringing of the ears?

A That depends on whether a cause can be found. Tinnitus, or ringing or other noises in the ear, can result from almost any ear problem, from infection to hardened earwax. Rarely, it can stem from an acoustic neuroma—a benign tumor of the acoustic nerve—or from Ménière's syndrome, an inner-ear disorder characterized by ringing, reduced hearing, and dizziness. Several drugs may also bring on ringing, namely high doses of aspirin or ibuprofen (*Advil*, *Motrin*, and generic) and certain antibiotics and antihypertensive drugs. In those cases, treating the underlying condition or adjusting the medication may silence the noise. In the vast majority of cases, though, no treatable cause is found. Playing background music can help distract you from mild tinnitus. Avoiding alcohol, caffeine, nicotine, and loud noises may also help.

EAR OF FLYING

Q Whenever I fly, I chew gum and yawn on both ascent and descent. Still, I experience pain in my ears, especially on descent. Afterward, my ears feel "blocked" for the rest of the day. Is there anything I can do about this?

A Your problem probably stems from congestion blocking the eustachian tube, which connects your nose and middle ear. When that happens, the change in cabin pressure during takeoff and landing can make the eardrum retract or expand, causing pain and impairing hearing. To keep the eustachian tube open, try taking a decongestant—preferably a short-acting nasal spray or drops, such as phenylephrine 0.5% (*Neo-Synephrine Regular Strength*, *Vicks Sinex*, and generic) shortly before takeoff. A second dose may be needed shortly before landing.

SWAB OUT EAR WAX?

Q *I use cotton swabs to clean wax out of my ears. But the box label warns me not to. What's the harm?*

A Swabbing out the wax can irritate or injure the delicate lining of the ear canal, causing itchiness or bleeding and increasing the risk of ear infection. If you have lots of wax, swabs can push it deeper into the ear canal, where it compacts and hardens. That can cause hearing loss, dizziness, or pain. Moreover, poking anything into your ear canal can damage the eardrum. Actually, most people don't need to clean out the wax, which gradually works its way out of the ear on its own. If it does become necessary to remove it, use ear drops such as carbamide peroxide (*Debrox Drops, E.R.O. Drops,* and generic); or even a couple of drops of docusate sodium (*Colace* and generic), a liquid laxative, or consider trying the following home recipe: Mix half a teaspoon of baking soda in 2 ounces of warm water and pour into a dropper bottle. Use a few drops twice a day for up to a week, and discard any leftover solution. (Don't use ear drops if you have a perforated eardrum or are prone to ear infections.)

Eye care

PLASTIC SUNGLASSES

Q *I've read that even clear plastic sunglass lenses block most ultraviolet light. Does that mean that my clear plastic prescription eyeglasses provide all the UV protection I need?*

A Probably. Only people who are at high risk of developing eye damage need to wear lenses with a special coating that blocks additional ultraviolet light. This includes people who spend large amounts of time in the sun; those who have had cataracts removed without the insertion of an artificial lens; and those who take certain medications, such as allopurinol (*Lopurin, Zyloprim,* and generic), psoralen drugs (*Oxsoralen-Ultra, Trisoralen,* and generic), tretinoin (*Renova, Retin-A,* and generic), or the antibiotics doxycycline or tetracycline.

SPOTS BEFORE YOUR EYES

Q *My husband, who is 69 years old, has a large gray floater in his left eye. Are there any medications or herbs that will dissolve the floater, or is there an operation that can remove it?*

A No. Floaters are tiny condensations in the vitreous, the jellylike substance inside the eye; they appear as tiny clumps or strands that float in the field of vision. The most common cause of floaters is the aging process, which can cause the vitreous to shrink and pull away from the retina, the light-sensitive layer at the back of the eye. A blow to the head can also separate the vitreous from the retina, allowing the unanchored jelly to shrink. While some floaters last for years, many fade with time and become more tolerable. Your husband could try repeatedly moving his eyes around, to shake up the vitreous and possibly push the floater out of his field of vision. Note that in rare cases, the retina may tear as the vitreous pulls away. So anyone who experiences a sudden increase in the number of floaters, particularly if they're accompanied by sudden flashes of light, should see an ophthalmologist.

FLASHBULB SAFETY

Q *Can flash photography injure a newborn baby's eyes?*

A No. Camera-light flashes last only a fraction of a second. That's too little time to damage anyone's eyes, even if he or she is looking right at the flash or having multiple photos taken. Further, the eyes can adjust rapidly to greater changes in light intensity, such as stepping from a dark room into full sunlight. Our consultants say that no special precautions are needed when photographing newborns.

VISION SUPPLEMENTS

Q *Can antioxidant supplements for the eyes fight macular degeneration?*

A Possibly, if you already have the potentially blinding condition but it's not too advanced. In a government study of 4,757 people, those with moderate macular degeneration who took a daily antioxidant eye supplement (*Ocuvite PreserVision* and others) reduced their risk of further retinal damage by 25 percent. But talk with your ophthalmologist first, since high doses of some antioxidants in the pills have been linked to health risks: beta-carotene with lung cancer in smokers, for example, and vitamin E with heart failure in people with diabetes.

EYELID CHOLESTEROL DEPOSITS

Q *I have cholesterol deposits in my eyelids. What causes them and how can I get rid of them?*

A These bumps form when surplus cholesterol in the blood collects under the skin surrounding the eyes. While they usually appear spontaneously for no apparent reason, they can also be a warning sign of high cholesterol levels, so you should have your levels checked. Regardless of the cause, the deposits are not harmful. But if they bother you, you can have them removed by a simple surgical procedure.

COMPUTER-VISION SYNDROME

Q *I spend most days working at a computer. Lately it looks as if there are more red blood vessels in the whites of my eyes. Is that normal?*

A Yes. The strain of prolonged staring at a computer monitor can cause those blood vessels to become engorged, creating the illusion that new ones have appeared. Your eyes may also feel dry and itchy. Resting, drinking plenty of water, and reducing eyestrain should resolve the problem. (Consult an ophthalmologist if the symptoms persist.) Here's how to help prevent the problem from recurring:

• Give your eyes regular breaks. And try to blink frequently, to distribute moisture to your corneas.

• Reduce glare by adjusting the surrounding light and the screen contrast or by using a screen filter. Keep the top of your monitor at or just below eye level, and keep your eyes at the same distance from the screen as you would from a book.

• Be sure that eyeglasses or contacts fit well and are the correct prescription.

• Consider buying either a liquid-crystal-display (LCD) monitor or a regular monitor with a high "refresh rate," both of which ease eyestrain by flickering less than other monitors.

TWITCHING EYELID

Q *I have a fluttering eyelid, which I cannot control. It flutters several times a day for 10 to 20 seconds. What causes this, and is there anything I can do to stop it?*

A No one knows for sure what causes twitching of the eyelid. Some doctors believe that rest and stress reduction may help. Sometimes pressing on the twitchy area for a few seconds provides temporary relief. If it hasn't gone away after three or four weeks, though, consult an eye-care specialist. If a thorough examination uncovers no underlying cause and the twitching is particularly severe and persistent, you may want to ask about the possibility of injecting botulinum toxin *(Botox)* to certain muscles around the eyes to stop the twitching. There are risks, however, since *Botox* is a drug that temporarily paralyzes muscles. And some doctors think that would be overkill for patients with chronic, unremitting eyelid spasms.

OFF-THE-RACK GLASSES

Q *Now that I'm over 40, is there any reason why I shouldn't use ready-to-wear reading glasses?*

A Go right ahead, if they're comfortable. Store-bought reading glasses are perfectly safe—and they're quite inexpensive. Such glasses work fine for most people with presbyopia (farsightedness due to aging eyes). However, you may need to switch to customized prescription lenses if you notice signs of eyestrain, such as headaches or tired eyes. Be sure to have an eye examination every two years or so after age 45 to ensure that your eyes stay healthy.

WHERE'S THE RUB?

Q My contact-lens solution is labeled "no-rub," but the directions say to use it to rub the lenses. Do I rub or not?

A Definitely rub. Labels on soft-contact solutions marketed as "no-rub" often recommend a longer rinsing time than regular solutions, ostensibly to compensate for shortening or skipping the rubbing step, in which you wet the lens with solution and use your index finger to gently wipe away debris. But a recent study found that rinsing lenses with solution for 5 to 10 seconds, as several no-rub products recommend, doesn't remove significantly more build-up than rinsing them for 2 seconds. And rubbing the lenses removes more debris than any amount of rinsing alone. The Food and Drug Administration web site says the instruction to both rinse and rub lenses "has always been part of the no-rub consumer labeling"—which makes you wonder why manufacturers can call the products "no-rub" in the first place.

CONTACT-LENS INFECTIONS?

Q I recently read that keeping extended-wear contact lenses in place overnight leads to increased risk of infection. I have been keeping my lenses in for a week at a time. Is that unsafe?

A It may be. Studies suggest that extended-wear contact lens users are 10 to 15 times more likely than daily-wear users to develop corneal ulcers, which can become infected. In general, the risk increases with the length of time you wear your lenses, beginning with the first night's use. It is much safer to remove contact lenses daily, then clean and sterilize them each night.

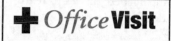

No silver bullet
for dry-eye syndrome

WITH R. LINSY FARRIS, M.D., M.P.H.

MY NEW PATIENT, A 52-YEAR-OLD CHURCH SECRETARY, SAID HER eyes had started to bother her about a year earlier. "At first it felt like something was in my left eye," she remembered. But now both eyes had become so irritated that her usual lifestyle was disrupted. She could not read for more than a few minutes at a stretch, and was no longer able to enjoy socializing or watching television.

At first she resorted to over-the-counter artificial tears. Driven by desperation, she was eventually using them about every hour or two. Her previous ophthalmologist had cauterized the ducts that normally drain tears from the lower lid into the nose, in hopes of enabling her eyes to retain more of her natural tears. The right duct had later reopened, but the procedure made little difference; both eyes continue to smart terribly. The doctor then prescribed cyclosporine (*Restasis*), a prescription eyedrop widely advertised on television as an effective treatment for dry eye, to no avail.

In the eye exam, I could see that the edges of her lower eyelids were filled with debris: mascara, secretions, and dust. Also, on testing, the film of tears on the surface of her eyes was unstable.

After she blinked, spreading the tears evenly over her eyes, dry spots appeared in about one-third of the normal time. The rest of the exam was normal. Her distance vision was an unsteady 20/20, only improving after blinking. As would be expected for someone her age, she needed glasses to read.

There was little doubt of the diagnosis: dry-eye syndrome.

The tale of tears

When people think of tears, they usually have in mind the reflex tears that well up when we're overcome with emotion, or when something gets in our eye. But the type of tear most important to the comfort and clarity of vision is the film that continuously coats the eye surface. It is a complex mixture of salt water, oils from meibomian glands in the lids, and dissolved mucins coming from small glands in the conjunctival tissues surrounding the eye. Any imbalance of those elements results in an incomplete and fragile tear film that breaks up and evaporates quickly.

Dry-eye syndrome can be a symptom of several underlying disorders, such as chronic eyelid infection or inflammation, allergic conjunctivitis, lacrimal gland atrophy, or several systemic diseases, such as Sjögren's syndrome and sarcoidosis. Turning immediately to artificial tears does nothing to fix those underlying causes. In fact, constant use of artificial tears washes away even more of the already fragile natural-tear film, and people can develop allergies to the preservatives.

Restasis was developed following the discovery of inflammatory products in tears. Its low concentration of cyclosporine has an anti-inflammatory effect. Additional therapies include other anti-inflammatory drops, including low-dose corticosteroids and allergy medications.

Clean, moist, and comfortable

Further testing established that the secretary had no underlying disease, allergy, or inflammation. I explained that no silver bullet would cure her misery overnight. Instead, we were going to try to help her natural-tear film repair itself. The first step was to discontinue artificial tears and prescription drops. Next, she was to make sure her living environment was maintained at 40 to 50 percent humidity (this required the purchase of a humidifier).

Most critical was a daily regimen of lid care. Twice a day, she was to wash her face with a cloth, then rinse the cloth with warm water and use it as a compress over her closed eyelids for 30 seconds. Next, she was to clean her lower lids with a dry, tightly wrapped cotton swab. This regimen accomplished three objectives: It removed lid-margin debris that was likely disrupting the tear film; gently massaged the meibomian glands in the lid margin so that they released oily secretions into the tear film; and stimulated the patient's own reflex tears.

At her follow-up visit three weeks later, she reported her symptoms had improved so much that she only had to use an occasional drop of artificial tears. Her lids were clean and her tear-film breakup time was in the normal range. We discussed the possibility of wearing glasses regularly, both to further retard the evaporation of her tears and to improve her overall vision. I recommended that she lower her computer screen so that by looking downward her upper lids would be lower and her tears would evaporate less. She smiled, and I knew we were on the right track.

Exercise and fitness

EXERCISE ENIGMA

Q *I've ratcheted up my exercise routine but I'm not losing any weight. What gives?*

A Several factors could be at play. You might have gained muscle, which can cause a slight increase in weight after a month or two of exercise since muscle weighs more than fat. In addition, some people simply lose weight faster than others. Also note that only aerobic forms of exercise—walking, cycling, or other activities that elevate your heart and breathing rates—burn enough calories to actually produce a loss in weight. (Strength training generally doesn't raise the heart rate enough to melt off pounds in the short term, though it definitely aids in long-term weight loss by raising your body's metabolic rate.) Finally, make sure your diet isn't sabotaging your efforts. While exercising might make you feel like you can eat anything you want, in fact it's very difficult to lose weight without also watching calories.

THE RISKS OF ANKLE WEIGHTS

Q *Is it OK to wear ankle weights during exercise if you have varicose veins?*

A No—but the reason has nothing to do with varicose veins. In fact, weights might help that condition by acting like compression stockings and by strengthening the leg muscles. However, ankle weights can put excessive strain on the knee and hip joints; that makes the weights generally inappropriate for aerobic workouts, regardless of the health of your veins. A better way to intensify such workouts is to gradually boost the pace or duration by no more than 10 percent per week.

EXERCISE AND METABOLISM RATE

Q *If I eat immediately after exercising, will I burn off more of the meal than I normally would?*

A Maybe. Physical activity of any kind speeds up your metabolism for several hours after a workout, depending on its intensity and duration. So your body is still burning calories at a faster rate during that time than if you hadn't exercised at all, a phenomenon that fitness aficionados call "afterburn." But the best way to boost the rate at which your body burns calories all the time—not just after exercise—is through strength training, which increases your body's ratio of muscle to fat. Aim for two sessions a week that work each of the major muscle groups, and use a resistance that allows you to do no more than eight to 12 repetitions of each exercise (or 10 to 15 reps for beginners or people with very little muscle).

MORE SWEAT, MORE GAIN?

Q *If I make myself sweat more during exercise, by turning up the heat or wearing more clothes, will I get more benefits?*

A Possibly, but it's not worth the risks. Exercising in a hot setting increases not only sweating but also heart rate and oxygen consumption. That increases aerobic benefits, burns more calories, and causes some immediate weight loss. But the steps you mention aren't recommended because they can prevent sweat from evaporating and thus cooling the body; that in turn might lead to muscle cramps, dizziness, dehydration, or heatstroke. And those rapidly lost pounds are almost entirely water; they'll return once you drink enough to replenish the lost fluids.

Advocates of forced sweating claim one other benefit: It removes waste products from your system and flushes impurities from the skin's pores. However, both effects are minor; normal bathing cleanses the pores better than sweating, and urinating eliminates far more of the other wastes.

MOTIONLESS MUSCLE GAIN?

Q *I've seen several ads for "no-work" exercise machines that stimulate muscles with electrical impulses. Can such devices help people bulk up or slim down?*

A No. The repeated shocks force rapid contractions, which can stimulate the growth of muscle fibers. But any gains are generally minuscule; even the best units, used to rehabilitate injured people, do little more than partially prevent muscle atrophy. Without regular exercise, electrical stimulation won't noticeably boost muscle size or strength, or burn enough calories to cause meaningful weight loss. And results from units like those you've seen advertised may be even more disappointing. A study of one popular model found that stimulating the major muscles of the arms, legs, and abdomen for 45 minutes three times a week for two months did not significantly change the participants' strength, weight, body fat, or overall appearance.

TIMING MEALS AND WORKOUTS

Q *Is it true that I'll get the maximum health benefit if I both exercise and eat my biggest meal in the morning?*

A That depends. For weight loss, morning workouts may be somewhat better. Some evidence suggests that exercising before breakfast burns more fat than later workouts, which are fueled mainly by proteins and carbohydrates from the day's earlier meals. (If you have heart disease, however, morning workouts may slightly increase your risk of heart attack.) Afternoons are probably better for building strength and endurance, since aerobic capacity, muscle strength, flexibility, coordination, and reaction time all peak between 4 and 7 p.m. But the most important consideration is to find a workout time that you enjoy, since that will help you make exercise a regular habit. As for your biggest meal, the timing doesn't really matter, with one exception: Stuffing yourself shortly before bedtime can lead to poorer sleep, since the body is still working hard to digest the food.

FITNESS VS. FATNESS

Q *I am attempting to better understand how to interpret the Body Mass Index (BMI). For example, suppose there are identical twin brothers, each 5 feet 11 inches tall and with the same body frame. One is a couch potato and weighs 178 pounds. The other is an athlete who engages in regular aerobic activity and weight training and weighs 185 pounds. The first twin, who is demonstrably less healthy, would have a BMI of 24.9 and be labeled "normal weight," according to current standards. The second twin, who is much healthier, would have a BMI of 25.9 and be labeled "overweight." Comment?*

A While BMI is a useful general weight guideline, it can be misleading when applied to an individual without considering other important attributes of wellness. Your first twin's sedentary lifestyle puts him at increased risk for cardiovascular disease despite his "normal" BMI. If your second twin is truly fit, with low body fat and high aerobic capacity, he has no reason for concern despite his slightly "overweight" BMI. The extra weight is probably just healthy muscle.

WHAT'S "PHYSICALLY FIT"?

Q *In a recent article you use the undefined term "physically fit." What does that mean?*

A It generally refers to cardiovascular fitness, or how effectively the heart and lungs supply oxygen to the muscles. While such fitness allows you to exercise longer—or just run for a bus without getting winded—its most important benefit is a reduced risk of major diseases such as coronary heart disease and stroke. Researchers evaluate cardiovascular fitness by measuring the heart rate during and after treadmill exercise. As a self-test, see how fast you can walk a mile without getting winded. That should take no more than about 18 minutes for moderately fit women in their 30s or 40s; the maximum for comparable men is about half a minute less. If you're past your 40s, allow an extra 30 seconds for each additional decade.

BEST EXERCISE FOR FAT LOSS

Q *I've heard that in order to burn fat, you must exercise moderately for at least 40 minutes, and that vigorous exercise burns sugar but not fat. Does that mean I should avoid high-intensity workouts if I want to lose weight?*

A Not necessarily. It's true that the body burns more fat than sugar during prolonged, easy-to-moderate exercise, but uses mainly sugar during hard exercise. However, researchers have not determined whether that physiological difference in fuel consumption translates into any meaningful difference in the amount of fat or weight you'd lose. What they do know is that you'll shed both fat and pounds if you consistently burn more calories than you take in from food. And the average person can do moderate exercise, such as brisk walking, for a much longer time than a vigorous one like running—and therefore burn significantly more calories overall. However, harder exercise can help you shed pounds if you use a special technique called interval training, in which you weave short bursts of vigorous exercise into a session of easier activity. Because the bursts generally don't cause much fatigue, you should still be able to exercise for a long time, and thus burn even more calories than if you stuck with a moderate pace only.

AEROBIC EXERCISE

Q Exactly what is it that makes an exercise "aerobic"?

A During aerobic exercises such as swimming, jogging, and cycling, the muscles demand a continuous supply of oxygen to burn the energy stored in their cells. That forces the body to improve its ability to use oxygen; this eventually benefits the lungs and heart by increasing the efficiency of breathing and pumping oxygenated blood. Strength-training exercise, on the other hand, is usually nonaerobic; that is, the muscles derive energy from biochemical reactions that don't depend on oxygen. However, such exercise is equally important and has complementary benefits.

AEROBIC CRAMPING

Q About 15 minutes into my aerobics class, my calves begin to cramp. Why does that happen, and how can I prevent it?

A Aerobic exercises, especially those that involve bouncing, tend to overwork the large muscle in the calf. The cramping problem might be avoided if you varied your exercise routine to stress different muscle groups.

Always be sure to stretch your calves before and after exercising:

Stand about two feet from a wall and place your hands against it. Bend one knee and move the other leg out behind you, keeping that heel on the floor. Lean forward until you feel the stretch in your calf. Hold that position for 30 seconds, then repeat with the opposite leg. You can also help prevent cramps by drinking plenty of water both before and during strenuous workouts.

REDUCING RESISTANCE

Q *A while back, you said that people get the maximum benefit from strength training by repeating a particular maneuver until they're too tired to do even one more repetition. I'm 74 years old. Is straining that hard appropriate for someone my age?*

A No. People younger than ages 50 to 60 (depending on their strength and health) should indeed pick a weight or other resistance that temporarily exhausts the involved muscles after 8 to 12 repetitions. But older individuals should reduce the resistance and do 10 to 15 reps. Moreover, they should stop when the exercise starts to feel somewhat hard but not very hard. (When you can exceed 15 reps without struggling, increase the load by about 5 percent.) Those precautions are needed because older people are more susceptible to muscle strains, joint injuries, and heart problems. While that lower-intensity regimen will yield somewhat smaller muscle gains, studies have shown that it can still reduce premature mortality by up to 50 percent.

SWIMMING FOR STRENGTH

Q *I swim a mile six days a week. I don't kick as hard as I'd like when swimming because it makes my back ache, so I exercise my legs by walking 5 miles once a week. Is this an adequate workout for upper- and lower-body strength?*

A The swimming gives your upper body a terrific workout. It tends to do less for your legs, especially if you don't work them hard. You might want to balance your upper- and lower-body workouts by swimming one day and walking the next.

ROWING MACHINES

Q *What are the benefits of exercising on a rowing machine?*

A This is one of the best ways to exercise your entire body. The sliding seat works your leg muscles, and the rowing action works the muscles in your arms, shoulders, and back. It's excellent for aerobic fitness and for building muscular strength and endurance. Rowing is also a very good way to burn calories and increase flexibility. However, since rowing involves a fair degree of back flexion, those with recurrent back problems should first check with their physician.

RESTING HEART RATE I

Q *What is considered a "healthy" resting heart rate for a 47-year-old man, and how much can an exercise program lower that rate?*

A A normal resting heart rate varies from person to person but is usually between 60 and 80 beats per minute, regardless of age or gender. With exercise and proper aerobic conditioning, however, the resting heart rate can be between 50 and 60 beats per minute. Highly trained athletes can have a resting heart rate as low as 40 beats per minute.

RESTING HEART RATE II

Q *I've heard that your resting heart rate indicates how aerobically fit you are, and that a rate below average means you're in good shape. But when should you take your pulse to determine that rate? Mine normally ranges from the upper 50s after waking to the mid-60s later in the day. When I'm tense and under pressure, my heart rate can soar into the upper 80s. Which of these is my resting heart rate?*

A The best time to determine your resting heart rate is before you get out of bed in the morning (unless you had a nightmare, which could make your pulse race). The resting heart rate for a well-conditioned adult is between 50 and 60 beats per minute. So your waking rate in the upper 50s is admirable. However, a heart rate lower than 50 in anyone other than a highly trained athlete could be caused by a problem involving the internal rhythmicity of the heart and should be checked.

WEIGHT LIFTING AND FAINTING

Q *While working out with weights, I suddenly felt weak and started sweating from head to toe. I feared a "silent heart attack," but my doctor checked me on a treadmill and said I was OK. What happened? I'd like to avoid a repeat.*

A You probably performed a so-called Valsalva maneuver when you were lifting weights: If you strain without exhaling, your blood pressure rises and your pulse drops. When you relax—as the weights are lowered—blood pressure can plunge and you're apt to feel faint. Proper breathing while you're lifting weights is essential. Before lifting, take a deep breath and then slowly exhale as you lift. The same warning applies to the use of weight machines.

Hair care

FEMALE HAIR LOSS

Q *Does the male hair-loss drug finasteride (Propecia) work for women?*

A It depends on the cause of the hair loss. Finasteride lowers levels of a male hormone that is the main cause of male-pattern baldness, or androgenetic alopecia. Women's hair loss can also stem from elevated androgens; in those cases, an off-label prescription for finasteride might increase hair density. But it's unlikely to help female hair loss from other causes, such as aging, genes, menopause-related changes in estrogen levels, drug side effects, vitamin deficiencies, or autoimmune disorders. And it's unsafe for women who are or may become pregnant or who have liver problems. Topical minoxidil (*Rogaine* and generic) is the only drug approved by the Food and Drug Administration for female hair loss.

FLAKE-FIGHTING SHAMPOOS

Q *Which shampoo is best for stopping dandruff?*

A It varies by person, since different shampoos target different causes of dandruff. As a first choice, try a product containing pyrithione zinc (*Head & Shoulders* and generic) or selenium sulfide (*Selsun Blue* and generic), which attack excessive skin growth on the scalp—a possible cause of dandruff—and are the least irritating to the skin. If that doesn't help, consider a shampoo with ketoconazole

(*Nizoral A-D* and generic), which combats the fungus P. ovale, another potential source of dandruff. If the problem doesn't improve after about two weeks, try a more potent, exfoliating shampoo containing sulfur (*Maximum Strength Meted, Sulfoam,* and generic) or salicylic acid (*P&S, Scalpicin, X-Seb,* and generic), which can help loosen up and clear away dead, flaky skin.

HAIR TODAY, GONE TOMORROW

Q *Is there a safe way to remove unwanted hair permanently?*

A Electrolysis is the only technique for permanent hair removal. A fine needle inserted into the hair follicle delivers an electrical impulse that kills the hair root.

Even the most skillful electrologist can have problems with the technique. Applying too much electrical stimulation can scar the tissue around the hair follicle. Too little can fail to destroy the root. Rather than risk scarring, it's better to err on the side of understimulation and repeat the procedure if necessary. However, doing so can become a prolonged, expensive process.

VITAMIN A AND HAIR LOSS

Q *I'm a 42-year-old man with thinning hair. I've read that too much vitamin A can cause hair loss. Since I eat large amounts of vegetables that are high in vitamin A, could that be partly responsible for my problem?*

A That's highly unlikely. While you could eventually suffer hair loss and other ill effects from taking supplemental megadoses of vitamin A, it's virtually impossible to overdose on the vitamin through the foods you eat. That's because the vitamin A in foods is mostly in the form of certain carotenoids—nontoxic vitamin-A precursors such as beta-carotene. Consuming large amounts of carotenoids can tint your skin orange. But that's not at all harmful, and it's reversible.

Thinning hair in a man your age is most likely due to male-pattern baldness, an inherited trait. Your physician can rule out other, uncommon causes of hair loss, such as an infection.

HAIR WOES

Q *The hair on my head is thinning while the hair in my ears is growing thicker. Why?*

A Hair loss in men and women is often hereditary, and it becomes more common with age. But even as hair thins on the head, changes in hormone levels cause it to grow faster in other spots, notably the ears, nose, and eyebrows for men and the face for women. Men distressed by hair loss can try the prescription pill finasteride (*Propecia*); our readers rated it first among hair-loss treatments in a recent survey. Topical minoxidil (*Rogaine* and generic) is available over-the-counter, but had lower rates of success among both men and women. Eating a healthy diet and avoiding blow-dryers and tight hairstyles might help slow hair loss. As for the extra hair where you probably don't want it, your best bet might be to buy a set of nose- or ear-hair trimmers.

Headaches

ICE-CREAM HEADACHE

Q *What causes the brief but excruciating headache you get when you eat ice cream too fast?*

A Sudden, intense facial pain can follow the application of any ice-cold substance to the back of the mouth and the upper part of the throat. Apparently, cold triggers a reflex spasm of the blood vessels there. The pain may result from interrupted blood flow to the tissues. Similar pain can occur in subzero temperatures.

PREVENTING HANGOVERS

Q *What causes hangovers, and can anything help ease or prevent them?*

A Alcohol can cause dehydration and disrupt cell function throughout the body, making you feel sick, or hungover, when any intoxication wears off. The amount needed to trigger a hangover depends partly on how much you're used to drinking: As little as one or two glasses of wine, for example, can leave some people feeling wiped out if they seldom drink at all. Of course, the best way to avoid a hangover—and to avoid getting dangerously tipsy—is simply not to drink heavily or more than usual. But several steps may possibly reduce the likelihood and severity of a hangover. Try not to drink on an empty stomach or when you're worn out from exercise or lack of sleep. After you've indulged, drinking lots of nonalcoholic liquids and popping a nonsteroidal anti-inflammatory drug such as aspirin or ibuprofen *(Advil, Motrin IB,* and generic) may be helpful, although it may upset a stomach already irritated by alcohol. Note that dark liquors including red wine are more likely to leave you hungover than lighter libations.

NOT TONIGHT—I'LL GET A HEADACHE

Q *I sometimes get a headache during sexual activity. Your report on special imaging tests mentioned that as one reason to see a doctor. Why?*

A To rule out the unlikely possibility of a brain tumor or aneurysm, which can cause headaches during certain types of exertion, such as coughing, bending over, straining during a bowel movement, or having sex. More likely, though, your headaches reflect muscle tension or vascular changes that occur as orgasm nears. "Benign sex headache," as it's called, most often strikes when the victim is tired, under stress, or having repeated intercourse. Some people first notice a dull ache at the back of the head.

If your headaches follow that pattern and a CT or MRI scan shows nothing wrong, you may be able to avoid trouble by taking a breather when you suspect an impending attack or by skipping sex during susceptible times. The prescription drug propranolol *(Inderal* and generic) can usually prevent sex headaches, but it can also diminish potency or impair orgasm. Some people are helped by migraine medications.

FEVERFEW FOR MIGRAINES

Q *I'm considering taking the herb feverfew to help prevent my migraines. Is there any good evidence that it works?*

A Yes. Some research suggests that supplements of feverfew may reduce migraine frequency and symptoms such as pain, nausea, and sensitivity to light and noise, but some evidence also suggests it's no better than a placebo. And analyses of feverfew products sold in the U.S. have found variations in their concentration and labeled dosage recommendations. Also, feverfew can block a key drug-metabolizing enzyme, leading to a potentially dangerous buildup in blood levels of numerous medications, and it may thin the blood, possibly adding to the effects of blood-thinning drugs. So if you take any medications at all, ask your doctor to check for potential interactions before taking feverfew.

✚ _Office_ Visit

Tracking down migraine triggers

WITH ORLY AVITZUR, M.D.

THE PETITE 23-YEAR-OLD ILLUSTRATOR HAD RECENTLY MOVED TO New York to start a promising job at an ad agency. She was clocking long hours at the computer, not getting enough sleep, and putting on weight due to a steady diet of takeout. When she began to miss work because of severe headaches, she was understandably worried.

She showed me her sketchpad of pastel drawings, which strikingly chronicled the visual auras—multicolored, jagged lights obscuring her left field of vision—that accompanied her headaches. By the time she called my office, the right-sided, excruciating, disabling headaches, often accompanied by nausea, were occurring up to three times a week and lasting hours on end.

Migraines affect 18 percent of women and 6 percent of men in the U.S. and are a leading cause of absenteeism and decreased productivity at work. The overall cost burden of migraines to society exceeds that of other chronic conditions, including asthma, depression, diabetes, and heart disease.

Although medications called triptans, such as rizatriptan (*Maxalt*) or sumatriptan (*Imitrex* and generic) can often halt a migraine in progress, nearly half of migraine sufferers who take those or other pain-relieving drugs are still dissatisfied with their ability to function or work afterward. And when used on a regular basis, over-the-counter and prescription pain relievers can paradoxically cause headaches, in essence converting sporadic migraines to chronic daily headaches.

It's obviously better to thwart the headaches from occurring in the first place, but quite a few commonly used preventive medications, such as amitriptyline or divalproex (*Depakote* and generic), might have unwelcome side effects, including weight gain and/or sedation. That might be why only 12 percent of migraine patients take them.

Common culprits

There's a better and more satisfying approach to preventing migraines, which is to find and avoid the triggers that set them off. Surprisingly, research has shown that more than three-quarters of sufferers are ultimately able to identify such triggers.

Beer, red wine, chocolate, and cheeses top the list for many. Hunger and odors are also cited, including perfume, which more commonly affects women than men. Many patients find that bright or fluorescent lights, the sun, or glare from TV or computer screens, particularly if flickering, can induce migraines. Insomnia has been shown to be related to morning migraines, and regular, but not too much, sleep is known to protect against attacks. Tension, irritability, and stress have long been linked to migraine episodes.

But it's not a precise exercise. Not all culprits cause migraines each time, and sometimes migraines result only when factors occur simultaneously—so-called "stacked triggers." For instance, while perfume alone might not cause a problem, drinking a glass of red wine might change those odds for the worse. To further complicate matters, some sufferers have a delayed response to stimuli, and triggers can even change over time.

Keep a diary

Because of inconsistencies, identifying a trigger might not be easy. Your physician might ask you to keep a headache diary—a log detailing your attacks and the medication responses—that can be reviewed over time. Those diaries can help patients and doctors identify possible triggers and assess treatment effectiveness. You should document each headache episode, describe its connection to meals and beverages, and note situational factors such as fatigue, sleep patterns, or stress. You should also list the medications you took, and write down how you felt afterward. Women should note their menstrual cycle as well.

If a trigger is a food or fragrance, simply avoiding the offending substance will do the trick. For light-related triggers, sunglasses or tinted glasses can be helpful. Behavioral therapies, such as biofeedback and meditation, are recommended when stress is a factor. Keeping to a regular sleep schedule can help with sleep-related headaches. Alas, some triggers, such as weather and time-zone changes, can't be easily manipulated.

The aura artist's headache diary was a success. It showed that certain food additives—particularly MSG, nitrites, and sulfites—prompted her attacks. She discovered that getting regular sleep and eliminating wine, Chinese food, hot dogs, and pizza significantly reduced her migraines. It took some time, but when I saw her six months later, she was headache-free, 20 pounds lighter, and back to sketching portraits.

Health fears and risks

RISKS AND BENEFITS OF GIVING BLOOD

Q *Are there any health benefits or risks to donating blood?*

A There are probably no benefits, except for the satisfaction of helping others, and the risks are minor. While some research suggests that giving blood might possibly help prevent cancer and heart disease by lowering the body's iron stores, that possibility is tenuous at best. And donating is generally safe, though it occasionally causes nausea, dizziness, or fainting. To minimize those risks, drink lots of fluids and avoid strenuous activity for several hours after donating.

NIGHT SWEATS

Q *I'm a 78-year-old man who experiences recurring night sweats. My doctor can't figure out why. What are the possible causes?*

A Several things besides the temperature of your bedroom can spark night sweats. Make sure your doctor has ruled out the most common causes: chronic infections such as tuberculosis, an infected heart valve, or AIDS; and tumors such as lymphomas and kidney or liver cancer. But not all causes are that serious. Using alcohol, aspirin, acetaminophen, or ibuprofen before bedtime can trigger sweating. (In women, night sweats are a common symptom of menopause.)

WHEN TETANUS THREATENS

Q *What sort of wounds would require me to get a tetanus shot?*

A Puncture wounds caused by nails, large splinters, animal bites, or anything else contaminated with rust, dirt, or animal waste or saliva are the most likely to become infected with tetanus bacteria. Infection can cause stiffness and spasms in the jaw, neck, and other muscles, difficulty breathing, and death. Fortunately, the odds of infection are minuscule if you've maintained your immunity with the recommended series of tetanus vaccinations: three inoculations before age 6, another about six years later, and booster shots every 10 years after that. However, since tetanus is very hard to treat, wounds that are especially deep or dirty may warrant a booster shot for extra protection if you haven't had one in the past five years. Note that the recent tetanus-vaccine shortage has ended, so if you're due for a booster, call your doctor.

SMOKING-CESSATION SAFETY

Q *I'm a heavy-smoking, overweight man who has had a hemorrhaged cerebral aneurysm [a rupture in an overstretched blood vessel in the brain]. To help me quit smoking, my doctor recommended a nicotine patch (NicoDerm CQ) plus bupropion (Zyban and generic) pills. Is that combination safe?*

A Possibly not. Wearing the patch helps wean you from cigarettes by providing a controlled dose of nicotine; bupropion reduces your craving for nicotine and the severity of any withdrawal symptoms. But the combination can cause blood pressure to rise, which potentially could cause a stroke. The two together are generally reserved for people who have a severe addiction to nicotine and haven't been able to quit with the help of either drug alone. Ask your doctor about starting with bupropion, and have your blood pressure checked frequently.

GERMS IN PUBLIC PLACES

Q Do germs on commonly used surfaces—like telephone receivers, ATM keypads, and bathroom door handles—pose a threat of infection?

A Yes, but the threat is extremely small. The relatively few bacteria and viruses harmful to humans can survive on dry surfaces for a while—typically several hours or days, but in a few cases for months or even years. Fortunately, the germs cannot multiply without nutrients or moisture. So even if they do manage to enter the body—through the eyes, nose, mouth, genitals, anus, or open wounds—there are usually so few of them that the immune system can wipe them out before any infection develops. To minimize this already minimal risk, wash your hands with soap and water; don't touch your mouth, eyes, or nose with dirty hands; and avoid obviously soiled or moist surfaces, where germs can multiply.

BLOOD SUGAR: HOW LOW IS LOW?

Q In your recent report on diabetes, you mention low blood sugar, but don't give an actual number for that condition. What's the threshold?

A Low blood sugar is technically defined as any value below 60 milligrams per deciliter of blood. But low blood sugar doesn't require treatment unless it's actually causing symptoms—sweating, palpitations, and hunger—which appear at variable levels below 60 mg in different individuals. People with symptomatic low blood sugar should be evaluated by an endocrinologist to determine the underlying cause.

FEAR OF FIBERGLASS

Q *The fiberglass insulation in my basement ceiling is exposed. Because my wife's throat sometimes feels scratchy when she works in the basement, she won't let the children play there for fear the fiberglass is harmful. Is it?*

A Probably not in this situation. Studies have shown a possible link between exposure to fiberglass and lung cancer, but only in workers who inhale huge amounts of the fibers for many years during manufacture or installation. Fiberglass insulation that is fixed in place usually doesn't give off airborne particles.

NORMAL BODY TEMPERATURE

Q *My temperature never seems to reach the "normal" level of 98.6°F. In fact, I rarely get a reading much higher than 97.5° or so, unless I'm sick. Is this unusual?*

A Not at all. The time-honored "normal" oral temperature of 98.6°F/37° C represented the average for healthy people, and that number has been revised downward to 98.2°F/36.8°C. Some perfectly healthy people never break 98.0°F/36.7°C. In addition, your normal body temperature can vary, depending in part on the time of day: It's consistently lowest in the morning and highest in the late afternoon or evening.

✚ *Office* **Visit**

Lyme disease: Beyond the rash

A FEW SUMMERS AGO I WAS CALLED TO THE EMERGENCY ROOM to see a 26-year-old graduate student who had collapsed in a local bookstore. He needed cardiopulmonary resuscitation in the ambulance on the way to the hospital. An electrocardiogram showed complete heart block, a potentially fatal condition in which the lower chambers of the organ beat independently of the upper chambers. The immediate insertion of a temporary pacemaker restored his heartbeat to normal. I later learned that he was a frequent hiker. He didn't recall a tick bite, but tests for Lyme disease were markedly positive.

Later that same summer I saw a 56-year-old dentist, an avid gardener, with pain in his left buttock that radiated down his leg to just below the knee, starting suddenly two weeks previously. His left leg was weak and his ankle reflex was decreased. An MRI of his lower spine was normal. I sent him to a savvy neurologist, who tested him for Lyme disease. He had it.

Lyme disease has been reported in every state in the U.S., with the Northeast, upper Midwest, and mid-Atlantic regions accounting for a vast majority of cases. It is caused by a bacterium, *borrelia burgdorferi*, transmitted by the bite of the minuscule deer tick. 30,000 confirmed cases were reported in 2009, easily making Lyme disease the most common insect-borne infection in the U.S.

Symptom smorgasbord

The disease has two distinct phases, early and late. The best-known early symptom, a bull's-eye rash, affects up to 80 percent of the victims. Other early symptoms include headaches, chills and fever, acute arthritis, and heart and spinal nerve-root problems. Late disease can include chronic arthritis, peripheral nerve injury, and brain and spinal cord symptoms.

The most common nerve complication is paralysis of the facial nerve, or Bell's palsy. The organism can also attack nerve roots adjacent to the spine, causing the kind of pain that afflicted the dentist.

Lyme disease affects the heart in up to 10 percent of people in whom the disease goes untreated. Symptoms can range from none to worrisome. Less often, it can affect the heart muscle itself or cause inflammation of the pericardium, or heart cover. Disturbances in heart rhythm can occur, but rarely as severe as in the graduate student's case.

Controversy has existed for years about the existence of chronic Lyme disease encephalopathy, or brain inflammation, that persists long after antibiotic treatment has erased all traces of the organism. People who think they have this condition complain of such vague symptoms as fatigue, memory loss, sleep problems, and an inability to concentrate. Blood and spinal fluid tests for Lyme are usually negative. Experts have yet to arrive at a definition of this syndrome, much less diagnostic criteria. But one thing is known: Repeated courses of intravenous antibiotics, plied by some self-styled "Lyme-literate" physicians, are useless and expensive.

When to look for Lyme

If you live in areas that harbor deer, deer ticks, and white-footed mice, see your doctor if you develop any of the following, even if you don't recall a tick bite:

- A rash resembling a target that expands over a few days.
- Flu-like symptoms outside of flu season.
- Acute arthritis (pain, swelling, warmth, and redness) of a large joint, usually a knee.
- Acute onset of pain along the course of a single nerve.
- Bell's palsy, or paralysis of one side of the face (rarely both).

- Erratic pulse, light-headedness, or chest pains (plus an abnormal electrocardiogram indicating problems with the conduction system, an abnormal heart rhythm, or evidence of inflammation of the heart cover).

The graduate student was treated with a month of daily intravenous injections of ceftriaxone (*Rocephin* and generic), a potent antibiotic. His heart block disappeared in a week, and the pacemaker was removed after a month. As for the dentist, his pain abated during a month's treatment with oral tetracycline. He has had no recurrences to date.

ALZHEIMER'S RISK

Q *Is there a natural way to reduce my risk of Alzheimer's?*

A Activity may slash your risk of Alzhemier's disease by 50 percent. That's the bottom line of a recent study of 716 adults in their 70s and 80s. Researchers monitored people's daily physical activity, including tasks like cooking and cleaning, for up to 10 days. People who were the least active were more than twice as likely to develop Alzheimer's disease during the next several years compared with those who were the most active.

Heartburn

HEARTBURN DRUGS FOREVER?

Q *I've taken esomeprazole (Nexium) for 10 years, though I'm not sure I still need it. Should I take a break?*

A Maybe. Esomeprazole and similar drugs, called proton pump inhibitors, treat heartburn and acid reflux. While some people need to take PPIs long-term for chronic heartburn, research suggests that many people stay on them for months or years without a clear medical reason. That's worrisome, since prolonged use might increase the risk of infections and fractures. Rather than stopping suddenly, which might lead to rebound heartburn, ask your doctor about tapering the dose.

SURGERY FOR HEARTBURN

Q *Should I consider surgery for my severe, chronic heartburn?*

A Only if all else fails: when lifestyle changes and drugs either don't provide relief or cause intolerable side effects. Surgery tightens the muscles that keep acid from entering the esophagus. But lifestyle changes plus drugs can reduce stomach acid enough to banish the burn, at least in the short run, just as effectively as surgery. Moreover, in one of the longest and best studies of such surgery, only one-third of patients remained heartburn-free a decade after having the surgery; the rest still needed to take drugs regularly to control their symptoms. And surgery is no more likely than drugs to prevent damage to the esophagus, which increases the risk of cancer.

Lifestyle steps include avoiding large meals and aggravating foods, not lying down right after eating, elevating the head of your bed, and stopping smoking. Heartburn drugs include antacids containing calcium carbonate, magnesium, or aluminum hydroxide, alone or in combination (*Maalox, Mylanta, Tums,* and generic); H2-blockers, such as nizatidine (*Axid, Axid AR,* and generic) and ranitidine (*Zantac, Zantac 150,* and generic); and proton pump inhibitors, such as lansoprazole (*Prevacid, Prevacid 24HR,* and generic) and omeprazole (*Prilosec, Prilosec OTC,* and generic).

HEARTBURN DRUGS AND LOST NUTRIENTS

Q *My mother takes lansoprazole (*Prevacid, Prevacid 24HR, *and generic), which eases chronic heartburn by reducing secretion of stomach acid. But I've heard that reduced stomach acid can contribute to nutritional deficiencies in older people. Should we be worried?*

A Possibly. Long-term studies have generally not shown any significant nutritional deficiencies in patients taking acid-reducing medications at any age, with the possible exception of vitamin B12 and magnesium. It's also known that aging itself can result in low vitamin B12 blood levels. This is due to loss of the cells that produce a factor that facilitates B12 absorption further down the intestine.

Liver disorders

GILBERT'S SYNDROME

Q *I was recently diagnosed with Gilbert's syndrome. My doctor says it's harmless. Is that true?*

A Yes—and it may actually provide some health benefits. Gilbert's syndrome increases the blood level of bilirubin, a yellow pigment in bile, by harmlessly reducing the liver's ability to dispose of the pigment. A potent antioxidant, bilirubin may help prevent cell damage and clogging of the arteries. Preliminary studies indicate that people with Gilbert's may have up to an 80 percent reduction in heart-disease risk. Other studies have linked high bilirubin levels with lower rates of cancer and heart attack, though only in men for unknown reasons.

TEST FOR LIVER DISEASE

Q *For several years, blood tests have shown that I have a slightly elevated level of the liver enzyme known as SGPT. But all of the other tests for liver disease have found nothing wrong with me. My doctor says it's not uncommon for a healthy person to have an elevated SGPT count. Is he right?*

A Most likely. In obese people it may be due to accumulation of fat in the liver. If you've tested negative for hepatitis A, B, and C, you have nothing to worry about. However, to be sure, your liver function should be retested periodically.

Medical procedures

LESS PAINFUL BLOOD DRAW

Q *My veins, which look adequate, are difficult to draw blood from, since they tend to roll. Is there anything I can do to make it easier and less painful?*

A Unfortunately, you're stuck with your troublesome veins, so there's little that can be done. An experienced, certified phlebotomist should know how to "anchor" rolling veins, so if you have blood drawn often, try to find one who can do it successfully every time. If you don't have a reliable phlebotomist, ask for an experienced technician and warn that person that your blood is "hard to get." Keeping your arm warm before the technician draws your blood may also help.

STRESS-TEST SAFETY

Q *I'm a healthy 74-year-old man who works out twice a week. During the exercise, my heart doesn't race and I have no trouble breathing, yet my doctor wants me to undergo an exercise stress test. Do the possible benefits of the test justify the risk that it might trigger a heart attack?*

A Exercise stress tests—in which an electrocardiogram (EKG) is taken during strenuous exertion, usually on a treadmill—can detect heart abnormalities that could make exercise dangerous unless you take special precautions. But like any physically demanding activity, the test does pose a very slight risk of heart attack. Further, it identifies only a minority of endangered people. And it sometimes finds apparent abnormalities that turn out, on further testing, to pose no real danger at all. So the test is generally worthwhile only for people who have experienced chest pain (especially during exercise), are sedentary and want to start exercising vigorously, or have either coronary heart disease or more than one risk factor for the disease (see page 145 for those risk factors).

LESS-PAINFUL BIOPSY

Q *I find biopsies of the prostate gland extremely painful. Your recent report on prostate cancer suggested using the topical anesthetic lidocaine to reduce the pain, but my urologist cannot figure out how that would be done. Please clarify.*

A Your urologist can apply lidocaine gel directly onto the rectal wall during a digital examination about 10 minutes before the procedure. That way the numbing effect can reduce the discomfort of both the entry of the probe and the cutting action of the biopsy itself. A recent study found that this approach significantly reduced the pain. (Note that many men do not find prostate biopsy extremely painful; the discomfort is often likened to that caused by a rubber band snapped against the skin; in addition, the biopsy site may ache after the procedure.)

NONINVASIVE ANGIOGRAPHY

Q *Your recent article on tests for heart disease discussed electron-beam computed tomography (EBCT) but didn't mention noninvasive angiography. Why not?*

A The two terms refer to the same procedure. Standard angiography, or cardiac catheterization, typically ordered after an exercise stress test reveals a potential coronary problem, is mildly invasive. Using a catheter snaked up into the coronary arteries, cardiologists inject dye to outline those vessels on an X-ray or computed tomography (CT) scan. That enables doctors to inspect the arteries for blockages. No dye is used in noninvasive angiography, or EBCT. Instead, a special CT scan measures the calcium buildup in the artery walls. Calcium is a major component of plaque deposits in the arteries, and levels of the mineral there correlate fairly well with the extent of the blockage. But EBCT doesn't provide the detailed coronary information that the stress test plus standard angiography does. And no one knows whether basing treatment decisions on calcium measurements alone is effective or wise. Our consultants say that EBCT has almost no role in treating people without symptoms of heart disease and limited use even in those with symptoms.

HEALTH CENTER SCREENINGS?

Q *A health center in my area offers a $3,000 "comprehensive physical" with scads of screening tests. Should I do it?*

A No. A number of health and "longevity" centers offer such packages, which include a battery of tests like whole-body CT scans, sonograms, and extensive blood work. The idea is that you can get a jump on treatment if the tests spot an as-yet-unnoticed disease, and peace of mind if they don't. But more screening isn't always better, and sometimes it's harmful. CT scans expose you to radiation and can yield false-positive results that lead to costly additional tests or biopsies—and a lot of needless worry. Further, detecting disease early doesn't necessarily lead to better outcomes; it may just expose you sooner to invasive procedures that pose risks of their own. In general, your doctor should order the screening tests for which there's solid evidence that the benefits outweigh the harm.

✚ *Office* **Visit**

Is that stress test really necessary?

THE 53-YEAR-OLD ACCOUNTANT, A LONGTIME PATIENT, WAS smiling when he came to see me for a routine exam after a winter in Florida. "I guess I'm going to live forever," he said. "My coronaries are clean." He told me that a golf buddy had persuaded him to get a checkup from a local cardiologist, something I never thought he needed because his health was good and he had no risk factors for cardiovascular disease.

Evidently, the Florida cardiologist didn't agree. He put the unquestioning accountant through what he called "routine" testing. That included an electrocardiogram and a stress echocardiogram (imaging of the heart by sonography before and after a standard treadmill exercise test). Apparently still not satisfied, the doctor ordered a four-hour nuclear stress test, in which a heart-seeking radioactive material is injected before and after exercise, and its eventual distribution in the heart muscles shown by a radiation detector. He concluded there was a problem. (It turned out the "problem" was an abnormality in the images caused by the patient's movement during the test.)

A day or two later the patient, by now convinced he was at death's door and would need open-heart surgery, found himself at a hospital, in a darkened X-ray room, undergoing a coronary angiogram. The procedure involves the insertion, usually into a groin artery, of a flexible tube that is threaded up into the heart. Dye is then injected to outline the coronary arteries and reveal any blockages. "When he told me that my arteries were clean, I was the happiest man in the world," my patient told me. "No matter that I wound up with bleeding in my groin, and unable to play golf for three weeks."

No symptoms, no need

The indications for cardiac screening tests for people without symptoms or a history of coronary disease haven't changed much through the years. The tests I just mentioned probably don't add much to diagnosis and treatment over and above what can be learned from knowing a person's risk factors.

Those risk factors are heredity (a parent or sibling who had a heart attack at an early age), smoking, hypertension, diabetes, elevated LDL cholesterol, low HDL cholesterol, lack of exercise, and possibly high triglycerides and obesity.

In fact, if you know most of those facts about yourself, you can enter them in our online risk-assessment tool, at *www. consumerreports.org/heartrisk*, to determine your overall risk for a heart attack during the next 10 years. You're considered high risk if you score above 20 percent and low if under 10 percent. Moderate risk is between 10 and 20 percent. Once you've figured out your risk factors, you should make every effort to modify the ones you can whether or not you have symptoms.

You might assume, as my patient did, that even if you have no symptoms, tests are still helpful because they will either reassure you or alert you to conditions you weren't aware of. But you shouldn't need a stress test to persuade you to improve your diet, give up smoking, and take your medication as prescribed. A stress test with normal results can create a false sense of security, which might cause you to relax your healthful habits. And an abnormal test might cause unnecessary worry and depression. Worse, it can lead to invasive and potentially harmful testing and treatment. You might even find yourself facing the business end of a scalpel with no more chance of preventing a heart attack or improving survival than what could be achieved with medication.

Some exceptions

That being said, there are a few situations that justify screening for coronary disease for people without symptoms. Those with two or more risk factors who are about to undergo complicated surgery or begin a vigorous exercise program might benefit from stress testing. And screening for those whose jobs affect other people's safety, such as bus drivers and airline pilots, could save lives.

I reviewed the tests imposed on the accountant but didn't have the heart to tell him that they were unnecessary, even if the outcome was a clean bill of heart health. And what a bill it was. But he remains convinced that "just knowing" made it all worthwhile.

Medications

PAIN RELIEVERS AND REYE'S SYNDROME

Q *Is there any evidence that over-the-counter pain relievers other than aspirin may contribute to the risk of developing Reye's syndrome in children?*

A No. Aspirin is the only analgesic shown to increase the risk of Reye's, a potentially fatal disease. But youngsters up to age 18 need to avoid aspirin only when they have a fever or a viral illness; the drug does not appear to cause Reye's syndrome at other times. Note that aspirin is a common ingredient in many cold and flu remedies. So youngsters' parents and adolescents themselves should check the labels for aspirin as well as its other names: acetylsalicylate, acetylsalicylic acid, salicylic acid, and salicylate.

EXPIRED DRUGS

Q *I try to buy vitamins and nonprescription drugs for my family in huge containers. But they often sit around for* *years, reaching their expiration date before we finish them. Would taking expired pills do us any harm?*

A Probably not, since they're unlikely to turn toxic. However, they might not supply the expected benefit, because all drugs and vitamins gradually break down and lose strength over time. The expiration date estimates when the potency will dwindle to about 90 or 95 percent of its original strength, under average conditions. Storage under ideal, manufacturer-recommended conditions—usually in a dry, cool place—can extend that date by about a year, possibly longer. Regardless of age, any drug or vitamin that shows signs of spoilage should be tossed out. Such signs include vinegary-smelling aspirin, crumbly tablets, sticky or melted capsules, or anything that has started to change color. Even without such signs, experts recommend discarding any drug or vitamin that's more than two years old.

LIVER-DAMAGING DRUGS

Q *In your recent article on the liver, you listed some drugs that can harm it. But you didn't mention the antifungals itraconazole (Sporanox and generic) and terbinafine (Lamisil and generic). Can't they threaten the liver, too?*

A Yes, along with many other drugs that are similarly less common than the ones we listed. The two antifungals––used to treat nail, skin, and systemic fungal infections—have recently been linked to several cases of liver failure, many of them fatal. As a result, the FDA now recommends that doctors order lab tests to confirm a fungal infection before prescribing either drug, and additional tests to rule out pre-existing liver disease before prescribing terbinafine tablets. (The cream and spray versions haven't caused such problems.) Patients taking either drug should immediately report any of these symptoms of liver problems to their doctor: persistent nausea, anorexia, fatigue, vomiting, right upper-abdominal pain, jaundice (yellowish complexion), dark urine, or pale stools. In addition, it appears that itraconazole can also damage the heart, so don't take the drug if you have congestive heart failure. Patients who develop any of the following heart-failure symptoms while on itraconazole should similarly consult their doctor: swelling in the feet, ankles, legs, or abdomen; severe indigestion; or extreme shortness of breath, especially when lying down.

NO-NAME ASPIRIN SAFETY

Q *Is it safe to buy no-name aspirin at a dollar store if it doesn't say where it was manufactured?*

A Probably, though it may be wiser to get your generic aspirin from a pharmacy or supermarket. Federal law requires that all over-the-counter drug labels provide an address for the company that packages or distributes the product. But even if that address is in the United States, the drug itself could have been manufactured anywhere on the planet. While we haven't heard any safety concerns about aspirin from dollar stores, *Consumer Reports* tests have raised questions about the quality of dollar-store brands of multivitamins, many of which failed to meet their label claims for certain nutrients or didn't dissolve properly. And since generic aspirin is inexpensive in general, you probably aren't saving much purchasing it at a dollar store.

WHEN TO USE ANTIBIOTIC SALVES

Q *Do I really need to apply antibiotic ointment every time I get a cut, scrape, or burn?*

A No, and sometimes it can actually be detrimental. For dirty wounds—those containing visible dirt or grit—applying antibiotic ointment is a good idea, since it sharply reduces the risk of infection, which occurs in about 20 to 30 percent of those wounds. But in clean wounds, the risk is only about 1 to 5 percent, so the drawbacks of the ointments can outweigh the benefits. In particular, allergic reactions occur in roughly 4 to 6 percent of people who use the antibiotic neomycin, found in *Mycitracin* and *Neosporin*, and 2 percent of those who use the antibiotic bacitracin, found in those ointments as well as some *Betadine* and *Polysporin* brands. Moreover, all antibiotics may contribute to the emergence of antibiotic-resistant strains of harmful bacteria. Whether or not you apply ointment to a minor cut, scrape, or burn, first wash the wound with soap and warm water to eliminate all visible grime and grit. If the injury is deep or extensive, rinse with water only, and seek medical attention right away.

SUPPLEMENTAL BLOOD THINNERS

Q *Each day I take 325 milligrams (mg) of aspirin, 2 mg of garlic oil, and 120 mg of ginkgo biloba. I take the aspirin as a blood thinner, but since the garlic and ginkgo have a similar effect, could I eliminate the aspirin?*

A If your doctor prescribed the aspirin to prevent or treat cardiovascular disease, definitely keep taking it. Aspirin is a potent, proven, and abundantly studied blood thinner or clot inhibitor. The possible anticlotting abilities of garlic and ginkgo have not been carefully studied, so the effects are unpredictable, and there are no dosage recommendations. If anything, abandon the supplements, since taking them together with aspirin may increase your risk of bleeding.

Men's health

PROSTATECTOMY AND INFERTILITY

Q *You recently said that after surgery for an enlarged prostate, virtually all men become infertile due to "retrograde ejaculation," in which semen travels up into the bladder. Aren't there ways to isolate semen from the urine for artificial insemination?*

A Yes. But the reliability of those techniques varies from person to person, depending on the viability of the sperm. Men who want to father a child after prostate surgery may want to consider storing sperm at a sperm bank before the operation. However, that's not a sure bet either, since freezing and thawing make sperm less vigorous.

PROSTATE SCREENING

Q *What is the PCA3 test, and is it worth having?*

A Preliminary evidence suggest that the test, known as Progensa PCA3 assay, might help determine the need for a repeat prostate biopsy if an initial one comes up negative. Approved by the Food and Drug Administration in February 2012, the test analyzes the cells in the first urine specimen passed after a digital rectal examination. A higher score suggests an increased likelihood of cancer, though the exact threshold hasn't yet been established. It might yield fewer false positives than the controversial PSA (prostate-specific antigen) test, but it might not be any better at detecting actual cases of cancer. Some evidence suggests that the PCA3 test might also help indicate the aggressiveness of prostate cancer in men who have it, but it hasn't been approved for that use.

VASECTOMY AND PROSTATE CANCER

Q *I am considering getting a vasectomy. But according to a release form for the procedure, "Some studies have suggested an increased risk of prostate cancer in men who have undergone vasectomy." Should I avoid the operation?*

A No. There's no plausible reason why vasectomy, which involves cutting and tying the tubes that carry sperm, would increase prostate-cancer risk. Men who undergo vasectomy tend to be health-conscious people who see their doctors frequently. So the higher cancer rate found in some studies probably just reflects better diagnosis of prostate cancer in those men, rather than any cancer-causing potential of the procedure itself. A review by the National Institutes of Health concluded that the overall evidence suggests no association between vasectomy and the cancer. The 20-minute procedure, typically done in a doctor's office under local anethesia, remains one of the most effective means of birth control, with an average reliability of 99 percent.

PROSTATE PROBLEMS

Q *Can urinary or sexual habits affect the incidence or severity of an enlarged prostate or any other prostate problems?*

A Those personal habits have nothing to do with the development of any prostate problems. However, modifying certain habits may help reduce the severity of symptoms. For example, urinating more frequently to keep the bladder from overfilling, allowing enough time to empty the bladder completely, and cutting back on fluids for several hours before bedtime can help reduce symptoms from an enlarged prostate. And since congestion in the prostate gland can aggravate the discomfort from chronic prostatitis (inflammation often due to bacterial infection), many urologists recommend frequent ejaculations to minimize that discomfort.

PUMPKIN SEEDS FOR PROSTATE RELIEF

Q *Can pumpkin seeds or herbal remedies reduce benign prostate enlargement?*

A Not likely. Limited evidence does suggest that the seeds may ease some symptoms of enlargement, including interrupted urine flow and a frequent, urgent need to urinate. But researchers suspect that the benefit, if genuine, stems from changes in the bladder, not the prostate gland.

Similarly scanty evidence suggests that two other herbal supplements, nettle root and pygeum bark, may possibly soothe mild symptoms. However, the best-studied herbal remedy for this problem is saw palmetto. Many small clinical trials have shown that it reduces symptoms. And one large trial found that a 320-milligram daily dose works as effectively in the short run as finasteride (*Proscar* and generic), a leading prescription drug.

At worst, pumpkin seeds are safe and nutritious, so there's no harm in trying moderate amounts for initial relief of mild symptoms. You might also try saw palmetto or the other herbs, though they can occasionally cause mild gastrointestinal distress, and there's no government oversight to ensure that the labeled dosage is accurate. For more severe or persistent symptoms, it's best to stick with conventional medications.

DOES SEX SOOTHE THE PROSTATE?

Q *My urologist says having sex frequently is good for benign enlargement or inflammation of the prostate gland. Is he right?*

A Possibly. Many men with those conditions report that ejaculation temporarily eases symptoms such as difficulty urinating and prostate pain. And one small study found that 14 of 18 sexually inactive men with prostatitis experienced at least moderate symptom relief after six months of ejaculating at least twice a week. One possible reason: Ejaculation stimulates muscles and nerves in the prostate region and eases pressure in the gland by releasing built-up semen. But while having sex or masturbating may possibly soothe symptoms, you should see a urologist to treat the underlying problem. For enlargement, treatment may include the herbal supplement saw palmetto; drugs such as doxazosin (*Cardura* and generic), finasteride (*Proscar* and generic), tamsulosin (*Flomax* and generic), or terazosin (*Hytrin* and generic); or in severe cases, surgery. A course of antibiotics may cure inflammation.

IMPOTENCE AND BLOOD-PRESSURE DRUGS

Q *The medication I take for high blood pressure is making me impotent. Is there a drug that can control my blood pressure without affecting my sex life?*

A All of the widely used types of blood-pressure drugs have been associated in varying degrees with impotence. However, two classes of antihypertensive drugs may be less likely to cause impotence. One is a group known as ACE inhibitors, such as captopril (*Capoten* and generic), enalapril (*Vasotec* and generic), and lisinopril (*Prinivil* and generic). The other group, called calcium-channel blockers, includes such drugs as diltiazem (*Cardizem* and generic), nicardipine (*Cardene* and generic), nifedipine (*Procardia* and generic), and verapamil (*Calan, Isoptin,* and generic). If your current medication can be safely changed to one of those without compromising blood-pressure control, switching may solve your problem. If not, your physician might consider prescribing one of the impotence drugs, such as sildenafil (*Viagra*).

PEYRONIE'S DISEASE

Q *What can you tell me about Peyronie's disease?*

A Peyronie's disease is a common disorder in which the penis becomes curved and distorted, especially when erect. The cause is unknown.

Local injections of steroids or calcium-channel blockers are sometimes successful. In carefully selected patients, surgery can sometimes be effective. It shouldn't be ruled out simply because of age. An experienced surgeon is necessary because of the possibility that surgery may create more scar tissue. When Peyronie's disease is combined with erectile dysfunction, the standard treatment is a penile implant. The recovery time for either procedure is about two weeks. Ask your doctor to refer you to a urologist experienced in treating this disease, or check the directory of the American Board of Medical Specialties, available at many libraries, and on the Internet at *www.abms.org* or *www.boardcertifieddocs.com,* for a list of board-certified specialists in your area.

Neurological problems

TAMING TREMORS

Q *I have essential tremor, which makes it hard for me to write. Is there any treatment for this condition?*

A There's no cure for essential tremor, which is the most common tremor disorder and may be genetically caused and can occur at any age, though it typically starts after age 40. However, daily doses of the beta-blocker propranolol (*Inderal* and generic) and the anticonvulsive drug primidone (*Mysoline* and generic)—taken alone or together—can reduce the intensity of tremors, typically by about half. Wrist-strengthening exercises can also help stabilize the hand, making it easier to write. In addition, try to avoid caffeine, certain asthma medications, oral decongestants, and stress, all of which can make the tremor worse.

SCIATICA AND NUMB TOES

Q *Last year I had sciatica from my back down to my right leg. The pain cleared up but left me with a kind of numbness in three toes (big toe and adjacent two) that I can't seem to shake. What can I do about this?*

A Your numbness probably stems from some chronic irritation of the sciatic nerve root as it leaves the spinal cord. This may be caused by a herniated, or "slipped," disk, a disk fragment, or a bone spur. Unfortunately, the longer the numbness lasts, the less likely it is to disappear. A consultation with a neurologist would be advisable.

SLAPPING GAIT

Q *What are the cause and treatment of "slap foot," which makes the front of the foot slap down noisily when walking?*

A Slap foot, or what doctors call a slapping gait, results when something goes wrong with the nerves controlling the muscles in front of the lower leg. The weakened muscles can't lift the forefoot, which hits the ground before the heel. The problem could be caused by a bulging or herniated intervertebral disk or a bone spur pressing on the spinal cord. It could also be caused by a damaged or inflamed nerve supplying the front part of the leg. Treatment depends on identifying the cause. If no treatment is effective, a brace can be helpful.

SHOULD I HAVE MY HEAD EXAMINED?

Q *I recently fell and hit my head while ice skating. I didn't black out, see stars, or have any other symptoms except for feeling slightly woozy for many days. Should I have gone to the emergency room?*

A Generally, that's necessary only if a minor blow to the head causes any of the following problems: a visible wound; classic signs of concussion, including loss of consciousness, disturbed vision, headache, stiff neck, nausea, confusion, or unsteady gait; or any symptoms that worsen in the days after the fall. In such cases a doctor will test your memory, concentration, and coordination, any of which may be impaired if the brain is damaged. Questionable findings may warrant a closer look with a CT scan or an MRI. Both exams can reveal signs of bleeding in the brain, which may require surgical drainage. (Resist taking anything but acetaminophen to squelch pain; aspirin, ibuprofen, and other anti-inflammatory drugs can increase bleeding and mask certain worsening symptoms.) Note that you're not out of the woods for 8 to 12 weeks. During that time, blood can collect under the covering of the brain, causing subtle symptoms such as balance problems or involuntary hand or foot movements. If so, drainage would also be required.

✚ *Office* **Visit**

The (not so) benign tremor

"AND I THOUGHT I HAD PARKINSON'S DISEASE!" THE 65-YEAR-old stock analyst exclaimed. Over the past six months her handwriting had deteriorated to the point that she was having difficulty signing checks. Since a good friend of hers had recently been diagnosed with Parkinson's disease, she feared the worst. I began to suspect her concern was groundless when I noticed that both her hands shook, and that she had a barely noticeable "to and fro" motion of her head—two signs that are uncommon in Parkinson's disease. And as she walked toward the examining room, her gait was normal and her arms swung freely—hardly the stiff-armed, hesitating walk so often seen with Parkinson's.

The exam turned up none of the other cardinal manifestations of Parkinson's—the typical masklike facial expression, the slowed, monotonous speech pattern, and the ratchety sensation the examiner feels when alternately flexing or extending the patient's arm. Moreover, her tremors seemed to worsen during the course of the examination, likely reflecting her anxiety, and failed to improve during purposeful movement such as touching her index finger to her nose. By contrast, Parkinson's produces a "resting" tremor (described as "pill-rolling") that tends to improve when performing a task. The diagnosis was unmistakable: She had essential tremor.

Tracking tremors

The cause of essential tremor remains a mystery, yet it's a common disorder that may affect as many as 10 million Americans. It typically begins after age 40 and often worsens despite attempts to suppress the symptoms. The limbs and body can shake severely enough to interfere with eating, dressing, and toileting. Essential tremor is often called benign in the sense that it is not a life-threatening disease. However, many people who have it consider it anything but benign. Some are forced into early retirement, and others grow so depressed they withdraw from active social life. The late Katharine Hepburn was a courageous exception; the actress continued to perform and have an active public life despite advanced and fairly severe essential tremor. Since many affected people have described similar problems in family members, physicians have presumed that the disorder is hereditary (our stock analyst managed to recall that her grandfather's hands "shook a bit"). Indeed, research has turned up two genes that may be responsible for the condition. There are no laboratory or imaging tests for essential tremor, so diagnosis has to be made entirely on clinical grounds and by selective testing in order to rule out other diseases that cause tremors. Those include advanced cancer and liver, lung, or kidney disease, which are usually all too obvious. Overactivity of the thyroid gland produces a fine hand tremor (in contrast to the coarse hand movements seen in essential tremor) and blood tests easily confirm that diagnosis.

Some drugs, including aminophylline, bupropion (*Wellbutrin, Zyban,* and generic), caffeine, dextroamphetamine (*Dexedrine* and generic), lithium, methylphenidate (*Ritalin* and generic), pseudoephedrine, and thyroid hormone can cause tremors. But, by and large, essential tremor has to be distinguished from Parkinson's disease, a progressive movement disorder caused by a neurotransmitter deficit in a certain part of the brain.

Treat that tremor

For mild essential tremor cases, treatment is available and can be helpful. A small amount of alcohol can diminish symptoms for an hour or two in three out of every four patients. Although that is not the ideal way to control the disorder on a long-term basis, it can come in handy at times.

The mainstay of treatment, and the only drug formally approved for that indication, is propranolol (*Inderal* and generic), a nonselective beta-blocker used to treat hypertension, chest pain, and migraine headaches. Some doctors prefer primidone (*Mysoline* and generic), an epilepsy drug also helpful in movement disorders. In addition, various tranquilizers and anti-anxiety drugs have been used, since the tremor tends to worsen in tension-producing situations.

Physical therapy, occupational therapy, and speech therapy should be tried, but results can be disappointing in severe cases.

The stock analyst's relief in learning she did not have Parkinson's disease was almost enough to improve her tremors. She has refused my offer to medicate her. However, she has taken to having a glass of wine with dinner. The only problem that continues to annoy her is getting the glass to her lips for that first sip.

✚ *Office* Visit

When nerves go on strike

A 54-YEAR-OLD FOREIGN DIPLOMAT WITH MILD TYPE 2 DIABETES was referred to me for painful neuropathy of both feet that was threatening to interfere with his career. His diabetes was well controlled through diet and metformin (*Glucophage* and generic), a drug that increases the ability of the body's cells to respond to insulin. He was also on moderate doses of gabapentin (*Neurontin* and generic), a drug commonly used off-label for the treatment of diabetic neuropathy, with only minor relief. To his dismay, he had been told he had an incurable disease and would have to live with it.

Neuropathies—disruptions in nerves that lead to pain, tingling, numbness, and sometimes even loss of function—are common yet often hard to pin down, and despite his seemingly forthright diagnosis, the diplomat's case was no exception.

His history struck me as inconsistent with diabetic neuropathy. His glucose control was nearly perfect, and his symptoms had come on rapidly over the course of only two months. Usually, diabetic neuropathy affects people with poor sugar control and develops slowly over the course of years. His blood tests were normal, except for a slightly low level of vitamin B12.

One nerve or many

Peripheral neuropathies involve one or more nerves after they leave the spinal cord or the brain. Notable examples of facial mononeuropathies are Bell's palsy, which results in paralysis of one side of the face (fortunately, temporary in most cases), and the less common, but very painful, tic douloureux.

Other mononeuropathies include carpal tunnel syndrome, which results in tingling and numbness of the palm and fingers due to compression of the median nerve as it tunnels under the carpal (wrist) ligament, and "Saturday night palsy," or wrist drop, which occurs from compression of the radial nerve (for example, by falling asleep at the bar with your head on the back of your wrists after a Saturday night of heavy drinking.)

And we have all hit our elbow's funny bone, which isn't so funny because of the pain and tingling in the pinky and fourth finger that inevitably follow. The guilty party is the ulnar nerve which lies unprotected at the outside bend of the elbow. Prolonged sitting with crossed legs can compress the peroneal nerve on the outside of the lower part of the knee, causing pins-and-needles sensations in that area. Occasionally foot drop, or the inability to flex the ankle, follows, and a brace may be needed.

The most common mononeuropathy—sciatica—probably has better name recognition than some presidential candidates. It results from pressure on the root of the nerve as it exits the spinal cord through a bony opening in the lower spine. That pressure can be from an osteoarthritic spur, a herniated (slipped) intervertebral disk or disk fragment, or spinal stenosis (bony overgrowth of the opening). Since the sciatic nerve supplies the entire leg, sciatica can cause aching and variable degrees of pain in the buttock, the back of the thigh, the outside of the lower leg, and the foot.

Polyneuropathies, as the name implies, occur when many small nerves are involved, commonly affecting the feet and less commonly the hands. The causes are numerous, including alcoholism, certain B vitamin deficiencies, excess vitamin B6, cancer, cancer chemotherapy, diabetes, hypothyroidism, chronic kidney disease, lupus, Lyme disease, heavy metal poisoning, rheumatoid arthritis, and certain viral infections.

Peripheral neuropathy treatments

As is the case with most complicated conditions, successful treatment of peripheral neuropathy depends on an accurate diagnosis of the underlying condition causing the pain. Unfortunately, in many cases the exact cause goes undiagnosed, and treatment is often just based on symptoms.

Topical products containing capsaicin or lidocaine may be of some help but are impractical for long-term use either because of the large area involved or because they lose their effect. Among the most prescribed of the oral medications are tricyclic antidepressants, such as amitriptyline, and newer anti-epilepsy drugs such as gabapentin—all used off-label. The evidence for those drugs is confusing and at times contradictory.

About the time we found the lowish B12 blood level in our diplomat, reports were beginning to filter through about metformin-associated B12 deficiency. He agreed to substitute another drug for the metformin. Within a few months his B12 level rose into the normal range. When I last saw him, his peripheral neuropathy had improved to the point that he no longer needed the gabapentin or any other pain medication.

Nondrug therapies—such as physical therapy, water therapy, massage, and vibratory or electrical stimulation—have not worked with any consistency.

✚ *Office* **Visit**

When you hit your head

WITH ORLY AVITZUR, M.D.

THE 47-YEAR-OLD HIGH SCHOOL TEACHER HIT HIS HEAD ON AN open locker door at the gym, but didn't think much of it. He was momentarily dazed and had a slight headache, though not enough to keep him from going ahead with his workout.

Ten minutes later, however, he became dizzy while lifting weights, and the friend who drove him home noticed that he seemed a bit confused. That night he began vomiting, and by the morning his headache had worsened. At his wife's urging he went to a hospital, where he had a CT scan of the head. It was normal, but the doctor discharged him with the diagnosis of a concussion and a referral to see a neurologist (me). His headache and dizziness had not improved when he showed up in my office three days later.

Every year more than a million people suffer head injuries serious enough to bring them to an emergency room, and an additional 235,000 are hospitalized. Eighty-five percent of these are concussions—injuries to the brain that result in a temporary loss of normal brain function.

Concussions happen when a moving object such as a soccer ball hits the head, or from direct strikes to the head from sports injuries, falls, assaults, motor-vehicle accidents—or a locker door. Our soft, gelatin-like brain tissue is usually cushioned by spinal fluid within the hard, bony skull. But an abrupt blow to the head or deceleration injury from a car accident, for example, can cause the brain to bounce against the inner wall of the skull and result in a concussion, essentially a temporary traumatic brain injury.

Is it a concussion?

The most typical complaints after a concussion are the ones my patient experienced: headache, dizziness, and nausea and vomiting. Concussions can also cause a loss of consciousness, amnesia, cognitive or memory problems, ringing in the ears, blurred vision, light sensitivity, and balance disturbance. If the complaints persist after the initial impact, it means the patient has developed a postconcussion syndrome that may also include restlessness, insomnia, irritability, and depression. Although most mild symptoms usually improve spontaneously within three to four days, they could last up to several weeks or even months if severe.

Because symptoms can differ from person to person and may be subtle, many people don't realize they've had a concussion. That can be particularly dangerous for athletes impatient to return to play, or for people who continue other risky activities while still having symptoms. They're at risk for second-impact syndrome, a rapid brain swelling that can occur when a second head injury closely follows the first one.

Even when the second blow seems minor, it can on rare occasions set off a chain of neurological events leading to death within minutes. Repeated concussions spread over months or years can also be dangerous. Researchers recently discovered that years later the injuries can cause a condition called chronic traumatic encephalopathy, which includes memory impairment similar to that seen with Alzheimer's disease.

Because of widespread criticism about allowing players with concussions to return to the field soon after being injured, the National Football League tightened guidelines last December. Formerly, players were allowed to get back in a game if they hadn't lost consciousness, but now they have to stay on the sidelines if they are having memory problems, dizziness, or a headache.

When to seek help

Anyone who has had a worrisome blow to the head should see a doctor for evaluation. It's especially urgent if symptoms include a loss of consciousness, a headache that won't go away, confusion, persistent dizziness, one-sided weakness, difficulty with language or speech, hearing loss, double vision, or visual loss. The exam is needed in part to check for more serious conditions, such as bleeding into or around the brain, that may require immediate treatment.

After a concussion, family members should observe patients for any changes in behavior or new neurological complaints. Most often the only treatment needed is over-the-counter analgesics such as acetaminophen (*Tylenol* and generic) or ibuprofen (*Advil, Motrin IB,* and generic) for headaches. In the rare cases where symptoms don't abate, a further workup is needed to exclude a blood clot on or in the brain. Fortunately, my patient didn't need that. It took some time and patience on his part, but when I saw him again several weeks later, he was fully recovered.

Nose, mouth, and throat disorders

EXTINGUISH BURNING MOUTH

Q *I'm a 45-year-old woman recently diagnosed with "burning mouth syndrome." Chewing gum eases the discomfort a little, and taking the drug nortriptyline helps somewhat more, but the pain in my mouth soon returns. What are the possible causes and cures?*

A Though the exact cause often remains a mystery, that syndrome—a persistent burning sensation with no visible irritation—sometimes results from the dry mouth occasionally associated with menopause. Chewing gum can help by stimulating saliva flow. Estrogen replacement therapy may also help restore the flow, but a burning mouth shouldn't be the only reason for taking the hormone. If estrogen therapy isn't an option, low doses of the anticonvulsant clonazepam can usually reduce the discomfort, by stimulating the release of pain-suppressing chemicals in the brain—although clonazepam itself sometimes adds to the dryness. When antidepressants such as nortriptyline help, psychological factors may be contributing to the syndrome. However, antidepressants may also dry the mouth; moreover, studies indicate that counseling reduces the pain more effectively than those drugs. Lastly, your doctor should check for underlying diseases or nutritional deficiencies that may occasionally spark a burning mouth.

Sore throat? Hold the antibiotics

"YOU MEAN YOU'RE NOT GOING TO PRESCRIBE AN ANTIBIOTIC?" The disappointed patient was a 50-year-old stockbroker who came to see me with a four-day history of sore throat, coughing, postnasal drip, and low-grade fever. He said that his previous physician had always given him a *Z-Pak* (a five-day course of the antibiotic azithromycin) for similar symptoms and that he always got better. I explained that it was more likely that he had a viral infection, for which an antibiotic would be useless. And I outlined some over-the-counter measures that might be of help. But he left the office in a huff, and I never saw him again.

Too much of a good thing

The age of antibiotics began in the 1930s with the introduction of sulfa drugs, followed by penicillin in 1941. In the last half-century, antibiotics have saved the lives of countless millions infected with deadly bacteria. The war against viruses, with a few notable exceptions, has not been as successful. Nonetheless, physicians began writing antibiotic prescriptions for many viral infections "just in case" bacteria might also be involved. Patients came to expect and even demand such treatment—like my stockbroker ex-patient. That's not good medicine. Unnecessary antibiotics not only expose patients to harmful side effects, such as debilitating diarrhea, but also lead directly to the emergence of resistant strains of bacteria that then go on to infect others.

In hospitals, at least 50 percent of antibiotic use is either unnecessary or inappropriate. In doctor's offices, where no one is keeping close track, the percentage may be even higher. Nowhere is this more evident than in the treatment of sore throats, which is one of the most common reasons adults and children visit their doctor's office. Even though it has been shown that a vast majority of sore throats are due to a variety of respiratory viruses such as adenovirus, respiratory syncytial virus, and rhinovirus, they are almost always treated with antibiotics.

Physicians probably overuse antibiotics for viral sore throats in part to appease miserable patients desperate for a quick cure. But the practice also dates back to a time when untreated sore throats were occasionally followed by rheumatic fever or acute kidney disease. Those complications developed from infections caused by the group A beta-hemolytic streptococcus—the infamous strep throat—that account for only 5 to 15 percent of all sore throats. The only other sore throat that can mimic strep throat (but with a negative throat culture) is that which occurs with infectious mononucleosis.

Virus or strep?

Today, there is no need to give antibiotics "just in case" it's strep. The organism can be reliably detected with a simple throat swab, with results available within 24 hours. But the disease can almost always be distinguished from a viral sore throat on clinical grounds alone. The patient is usually less than 50 years of age, and the sore throat comes on like gangbusters within hours or overnight, making swallowing so difficult that drooling can occur. The breath has a foul odor, and even speech is affected. A fever in excess of 101°F, accompanied by chilly sensations, is common, and you can easily feel tender swollen lymph nodes under the jaw. Inspection of the throat shows yellowish pus overlying the tonsils. Since group A strep evidently lacks the ingenuity to have developed resistance, penicillin is still the mainstay of treatment unless you're allergic to it.

Viral sore throats develop over the course of a few days and are invariably accompanied by a runny nose, postnasal drip, a cough with clear or greenish sputum, and a low-grade fever or no fever at all. No medicine will cure them. The only treatment is "tincture of time"—waiting out the one to two weeks it can take for symptoms to abate on their own. The flu (also a viral illness) has symptoms similar to a viral sore throat, except for more intense muscle aches and perhaps a higher fever, and is treatable with the antiviral drug oseltamivir (*Tamiflu*) if given early enough in the course of the illness.

You can manage symptoms with acetaminophen (*Tylenol* and generic), nasal sprays or drops, throat lozenges, and gargling with warm saltwater. Of course, there's always good old chicken soup, which, in my opinion, would have helped that stockbroker more than a whole carload of *Z-Paks*.

DOUSING DRY MOUTH

Q *I'm a 63-year-old woman who takes a daily multivitamin for general health, omeprazole (Prilosec, Prilosec OTC, and generic) for heartburn, and estrogen (Premarin) to relieve symptoms of menopause. Though I'm in good overall health and don't drink alcohol or smoke, I suffer from severe, chronic dry mouth. My dentist doesn't know what's causing it or how I could moisten my mouth. Do you?*

A This common condition is usually a side effect of drug therapy. Omeprazole sometimes does interfere with salivation—especially at high doses. So ask your doctor if you could try a lower dosage or switch to another medication to ease your heartburn without drying your mouth. The underlying cause could also be a medical condition such as Sjogren's syndrome, an often-undiagnosed autoimmune disorder, or one of several salivary-gland or neurological diseases.

If the cause can't be determined, treated, or modified, try stimulating your salivary glands by eating strong-tasting or fibrous foods (such as carrots and celery), sucking on sugar-free hard candy, or chewing sugar-free gum. (Since the saliva shortage raises the risk of cavities, limit your sugar intake and exercise good dental hygiene.) Sipping liquid frequently, sucking on ice cubes or sugar-free Popsicles, breathing through your nose, and using a humidifier can further help keep your mouth moist. If those steps fail, an over-the-counter saliva substitute (*Moi-Stir, Mouthkote, Optimoist, Salivart*) can provide short-term relief, and the prescription drug pilocarpine (*Salagen* and generic) may increase saliva output (though it's not suitable for people with certain chronic diseases).

TOO MUCH SALIVA

Q I salivate so much that the saliva chokes me when I try to sleep. My doctor hasn't been able to help. What could the problem be?

A It's possible that you just have trouble swallowing. That problem, which people often don't notice, can cause saliva to collect in your mouth, making you think your saliva glands are working overtime. An ear, nose, and throat specialist can test your swallowing reflex, which can be damaged by several neurologic or muscular disorders. If the reflex is normal, you should probably see a dentist who specializes in salivary-gland disorders—usually at a university medical center or large hospital—who can measure your saliva secretion. If excessive salivation is the problem, doctors should check for an underlying cause, such as a drug side effect, gastroesophageal reflux, or a rare effect of diabetes.

TOPOGRAPHICAL TONGUE

Q I have intermittent bouts of "geographica lingua," in which my tongue sheds tissue, creating deep grooves that make eating uncomfortable. What causes this and what can I do about it?

A Unfortunately, the cause and cure are both unknown. But you may be able to ease the mild discomfort of this otherwise harmless, relatively uncommon condition. Since the grooves tend to develop around points of irritation, avoid brushing your tongue or moving it around excessively. And have your dentist smooth any rough or sharp edges on your teeth and fix any ill-fitting dental appliances.

OVERREACTIVE NOSE

Q *After enduring a stuffy nose for almost a year, I was diagnosed with vasomotor rhinitis, a nonallergic condition. My allergist told me that anger can aggravate it, but there's no cure. Is that true?*

A Yes. This common condition occurs when blood vessels in the nose overreact to certain environmental or emotional stimuli by swelling up and triggering excess mucus production. Common culprits include changes in air temperature and humidity, strong odors, spicy food, and even strong feelings like anger. If you can identify the triggers, you may be able to neutralize or avoid them. Exercising and keeping a hostility diary, for example, may curb anger. Although drugs cannot completely relieve symptoms, your doctor may prescribe an oral decongestant, an antihistamine, or a steroid nasal spray that can provide limited relief. Avoid over-the-counter decongestant nasal sprays, such as *Afrin* or *Otrivin*, which can actually make matters worse.

WINTER NOSEBLEEDS

Q *I frequently get nosebleeds in the winter. What's the best way to stop then?*

A Most nosebleeds occur just inside the nostrils and can be stopped by tilting your head forward slightly and pinching the soft area of your nose. Holding a cold compress over the bridge of your nose during or after a nosebleed might also help. Those that start farther back in the nose are less common but more serious, since they might not respond to compression with your fingers. If bleeding lasts longer than 20 minutes, head to an emergency room for treatment. Don't put gauze or other materials inside your nose, which could disturb clotting and cause bleeding to restart when you remove it. And use a room humidifier (ideally set to 30 or 50 percent humidity), since winter nosebleeds often stem from dry indoor air.

THRUSH

Q *A few months ago I developed "thrush"—whitish patches on my tongue and on the back of my throat—after a six-day course of intravenous antibiotics. The antibiotics apparently killed the normal protective bacteria in my mouth, allowing the thrush to develop. Now I'm concerned about my intestinal bacteria as well. So I've been taking L. acidophilus and bifidus supplements to reestablish those bacteria. Is that the right thing to do?*

A No. The bacterial imbalance that follows use of antibiotics may indeed allow other bacteria or fungi to take hold. Those include the candida that cause thrush. But while the "intestinal flora" supplements you mention have shown some benefits at reducing antibiotic-associated diarrhea, they have not been shown to be very effective at treating thrush. You should treat the candida with an effective antifungal medicine, such as oral fluconazole (*Diflucan* and generic) or nystatin (*Nilstat*). The usual bacterial population will return to your mouth and intestinal tract on its own.

SMELL LOSS

Q *I'm 83 years old and seem to be losing my ability to smell. My doctor says I should travel nearly 100 miles for special smell tests. Is loss of smell really such a significant problem?*

A It might be, since it could affect your health and safety. You may be unable to detect smoke or gas in your home or realize when food has spoiled. And your nose is largely responsible for your sense of taste. Loss of taste could cause you to use excessive salt or sugar in hopes of increasing flavor, or to lose interest in eating entirely. And it could signal an underlying disorder such as vitamin-B12 or folic-acid deficiency, hypothyroidism, diabetes, Parkinson's disease, stroke, or a brain tumor.

But you probably don't have to take special tests to evaluate your loss of smell. Instead, you can confirm it at home: Close your eyes and see if you can distinguish chocolate ice cream from vanilla, or one jelly-bean flavor from another. Or douse a cloth with alcohol and see if you can smell it while slowly bringing the cloth from your chest up to your nose.

If you flunk those tests, or if food seems generally tasteless, ask your doctor to rule out any underlying medical problems. Loss of smell could also be a medication side effect; if so, adjusting the dosage or switching to a different drug can help.

If the problem persists, be extra careful about turning off the gas range, have someone check for gas leaks and food spoilage, and make sure your home has functioning gas and smoke detectors. Choosing spicy flavors and interesting textures can help keep food tasty.

LOSS OF TASTE AND SMELL

Q *At the age of 54, I seem to be losing my sense of taste and smell. What might be causing this?*

A Like hearing and vision, taste and smell tend to deteriorate with age. In addition, various illnesses and injuries can damage the nerves connecting the sense organs to the brain. Loss of smell, for example, can be caused by nasal or sinus infections, nasal polyps, meningitis, or brain tumors. Loss of smell can affect taste. So can allergies, tongue injuries, stroke, or tumors. You should consult your physician to rule out possible underlying disorders.

POSTNASAL DRIP

Q *I suffer from postnasal drip, which constantly fills my throat with phlegm. What can I do about it?*

A Probably not much. Postnasal drip is typically caused by air pollution, allergies, or infections. The irritated membranes in your nose and sinuses thicken and produce too much mucus. When the condition becomes chronic, it's often difficult to tell what caused it. And it's seldom cured.

Side effects from the standard medications used for postnasal drip—antibiotics, antihistamines, and decongestants—often outweigh their meager benefits. If you should try those drugs and they don't work, see an otorhinolaryngologist (ear, nose, and throat specialist). Once cysts, polyps, and tumors have been ruled out, either a corticosteroid nasal spray or cortisone injections into the nasal membranes may help.

TOUGH PILL TO GET DOWN

Q *I've recently become unable to swallow pills of any size. What could cause that?*

A It depends on whether the problem is limited to medications. Some people have an unexplained inability to swallow pills or tablets, but no problems swallowing anything else. If that's the case, you might talk with your doctor about switching to chewable, dissolvable, or liquid versions of your medications. Trouble swallowing in general can stem from several causes, including acid reflux or a narrowing of the esophagus from something as benign as a stuck piece of food or as serious as a cancerous tumor. If trouble swallowing occurs regularly or is accompanied by choking, pain, vomiting, or weight loss, see your doctor to determine the cause.

✚ *Office* **Visit**

A tough one to swallow

"I THOUGHT IT WAS ABOUT TIME I LOOKED INTO THIS," SAID A 49-year-old politician, an infrequent seeker of medical attention. His complaint of pain while swallowing had been present on and off for a number of years. "Since it mostly bothered me during campaign time, especially at fund-raising affairs when I had to make after-dinner speeches, I never thought it was important enough to mention; probably just tension and stress." But some publicity about cancer of the esophagus raised his medical consciousness enough to make him schedule an office visit.

Swallowing is a natural action that we perform over a hundred times a day without giving it a second thought, but it's actually a complicated maneuver involving the coordinated actions of nerves and muscles of the tongue, throat, and esophagus. When everything is working right, people can swallow even while standing on their heads, but even a minor glitch in any of those systems can throw the process off enough for them to notice.

Discomfort, disability, or pain during the act of swallowing (dysphagia), especially when persistent or recurrent, should be brought to medical attention because it almost always signifies some abnormality. The question is: Which one?

FINDING A CAUSE

Difficulty in starting the swallowing process arises from damage to the nerves and muscles in the back of the throat. A stroke is the most common cause but is usually accompanied by other symptoms, such as weakness in an arm or leg. My patient had no symptoms suggestive of a stroke, and besides, stroke-related swallowing problems don't usually produce the pain that he complained of.

Nor, after listening carefully to his story, did I think he had esophageal cancer, the concern that had led him to my office in the first place. Dysphagia caused by this usually aggressive malignancy gets rapidly worse and is invariably accompanied by weight loss. His symptoms were intermittent and hadn't gotten any worse over several years.

He didn't have heartburn, often caused by the reflux of stomach acid up into the esophagus. Chronic acid reflux can irritate or ulcerate the esophagus enough to interfere with swallowing. Besides, he had already tried myriad over-the-counter antacid pills and liquids, none of which had done him any good. If he had had heartburn, those should have at least moderated his symptoms.

He didn't take any of the medications known to produce a little-known condition called "pill dysphagia," difficulty in swallowing due to drugs capable of causing inflammation and eventual narrowing or stricture of the lower esophagus. Most cases of pill dysphagia arise from antibiotics, notably doxycycline (*Vibramycin* and generic). Other pills commonly involved in pill dysphagia are potassium tablets, aspirin, and nonsteroidal anti-inflammatory medications such as ibuprofen (*Advil*, *Motrin*, and generic), corticosteroids such as prednisone (*Deltasone*, *Orasone*, and generic), and the heart drug quinidine (*Cardioquin* and generic).

Finally, there was nothing in his history to suggest that he had infectious esophagitis. This inflammation of the esophagus is usually caused by a fungal infection in someone whose immune system has been compromised, for example, by immunosuppressive drugs (after, say, a kidney transplant), HIV infection, or a prolonged course of antibiotics or corticosteroids. He didn't fit into any of those categories.

PROBLEM SOLVED

I referred our politician to a gastroenterology colleague, who performed an upper endoscopy, in which the esophagus is viewed through a flexible lighted tube inserted into the mouth and then threaded into the esophagus. In the lower-most part of the esophagus, he saw a ring-shaped web of the esophageal lining projecting into the passageway.

This proved to be a Schatzki's ring: a benign, fleshy protrusion capable of retarding the passage of solid foods from the lower end of the esophagus into the stomach. Believed by some to be congenital, a Schatzki's ring can produce obstructive symptoms such as pain or discomfort while swallowing solid food, particularly meat (hence its nickname: "steakhouse syndrome"). The condition occurs in about 15 percent of people but causes symptoms in relatively few. No one knows why the symptoms come and go and show up only in later life—but they match my patient's story exactly.

The treatment was simple and immediate. At the same sitting, while the patient was still sedated, the gastroenterologist inserted a dilator tube that broke the web. That was more than two years ago, and the dysphagia has not returned.

Parenting and pregnancy

BUCKLE UP IF YOU'RE PREGNANT

Q *Is it safe for a woman to wear a safety belt while pregnant?*

A Yes. Studies have found that a properly worn safety belt not only helps protect the expectant mother during a car accident but also dramatically reduces the likelihood of harm to the fetus. Pregnant women using safety belts are half as likely as their unrestrained counterparts to go into premature labor or deliver a low-birthweight baby after an accident. The lower belt should fit under the woman's belly and snugly across her lap, with the upper portion running between her breasts. Whenever possible, pregnant women should ride as passengers, to avoid possible contact with the steering wheel during an accident. And everyone should leave airbags operational and keep their seat as far away as comfortably possible from the dashboard or steering wheel.

BREAST-FEEDING AND BRITTLE BONES

Q *Recently you said that breast-feeding may reduce the mother's risk of osteoporosis. Why is that? Doesn't secreting the milk cause a loss of calcium?*

A Yes it does. As a result, bone density typically does decline during the breast-feeding months. However, studies have found that breast-feeding does not increase the mother's risk of thin bones and fractures in later life. And, in fact, some studies show that breast-feeding actually decreases the risk. That's probably because calcium absorption from dietary sources increases after breast-feeding stops; as a result, women quickly regain the lost bone and wind up with even more than they had before.

POST-PILL PREGNANCY

Q Is it true that a woman should wait three months after discontinuing birth-control pills before getting pregnant? If so, why?

A It's a good idea to hold off trying to conceive for at least a month or two, to allow time for your menstrual periods to become regular. Irregular periods make it harder to detect ovulation and to determine your due date when you do become pregnant. However, we know of no evidence that becoming pregnant immediately after discontinuing birth-control pills causes harm to mother or child.

POSTPARTUM DEPRESSION

Q What causes postpartum depression? What are the latest treatments?

A Postpartum depression—not the more common postpartum "blues"—is a psychiatric disorder that can severely impair day-to-day functioning. Its onset is usually within the first few weeks or months after childbirth. A woman who has once had postpartum depression can experience it again after future births.

The causes of postpartum depression are not well understood. The sudden change from the pregnant state, with accompanying changes in hormone levels, probably plays some role. Occasionally postpartum depression can be part of a temporary inflammatory thyroid disease called thyroiditis.

In contrast to the self-limited "blues," which usually lasts only a short time and needs only emotional support, true postpartum depression requires the attention of a psychiatrist. Certain antidepressant medications can help. Rarely, electroconvulsive (electric shock) therapy may be necessary.

Respiratory infections

WHERE THERE'S SMOKE

Q *A year or so ago I was diagnosed as having a bronchial infection caused by* Hemophilus influenza *bacteria. Despite having taken three or four antibiotics, I still have a very productive cough. Could the fact that I smoke cigarettes be hampering my recovery?*

A Very likely. Not only do smokers experience more respiratory infections than nonsmokers do, but they also are likely to have more difficulty recovering. Smoking destroys cilia, the tiny filaments that help to move infected mucus up and out of the lungs. And the ability of the lungs to repair tissue damage is impaired by years of smoking.

ANTIBIOTICS FOR A BAD COLD

Q *I've had two particularly bad colds over the past year. Both times, my doctor prescribed antibiotics. I thought that a cold is a viral infection and that antibiotics aren't effective against viruses. Why the antibiotics?*

A That depends. Antibiotics indeed won't do anything for a viral infection such as the common cold. But sometimes a cold virus leads to a bacterial infection in the sinus or bronchial airways, which does require antibiotics. Sinus infections can produce a thick, yellow or deeply colored discharge from the nose, tenderness or pain just above or below the eyes, and mild fever. Bronchial infections can also cause fever as well as a cough that brings up greenish-yellow sputum or even some blood.

If you have none of those symptoms, you shouldn't take antibiotics. The drugs can cause such side effects as nausea, diarrhea, and rashes. They can also kill off the body's own protective bacteria, allowing fungal infections to grow, and inappropriate use can add to the growing and serious problem of antibiotic-resistant germs.

Skin care

MANICURES AND NAIL INFECTIONS

Q My nail salon uses the same set of tools on many different clients, disinfecting them between jobs. Is that enough to avoid spreading infections, or should I choose a salon that provides a separate set of tools for each client?

A That depends on how well they're cleaned. Most salons meticulously eliminate the risk of transmitting infection by properly sterilizing with either steam or a chemical disinfectant. If a salon is licensed and looks clean, and the technicians are fastidious, you probably don't have to worry. If you're unsure, ask about sterilization methods (an establishment that takes infection control seriously should be eager to tell you about it). If you're still skeptical, bring your own tools or find a salon that offers each client a separate set. Regardless of the tools used, avoid having your cuticles trimmed since that can promote infection. And contact your physician if your fingers burn, itch, sting, or turn red after a manicure—all signs of possible infection or allergic reaction.

DO SUNSCREENS EXPIRE?

Q *Should I throw away the tubes of sunscreen that have been sitting in my medicine cabinet for several years?*

A Most likely. Sunscreens eventually start losing their sun-protecting power when the ingredients start to separate. That generally happens after the expiration date, which should be printed on the label; it's usually two to three years after the product was made. Toss out any sunscreen that has expired or shows signs of separating, such as grittiness or changed appearance.

HYDROGEN PEROXIDE FOR CUTS

Q *I often see hydrogen peroxide listed among the recommended essentials for a medicine cabinet or first aid kit. Is it better for cuts than soap and water?*

A Usually not. Many people do use hydrogen peroxide, thinking it will help clean and kill germs in minor cuts and scratches. But studies that have tested it for that use have generally failed to show any benefit. Its bubbling action does appear to help remove debris from minor wounds, but soap and running water probably work just as well. And there's at least a theoretical risk that the solution can irritate sensitive skin. So you're probably better off using mild soap and clean water to decontaminate minor wounds, and consider hydrogen peroxide in situations where clean water isn't available, such as while hiking or camping.

ADULT ACNE

Q *Can any drugs, creams, or other products worsen my adult acne?*

A Yes—if it's really acne. In adults, that problem is usually caused by hormonal fluctuations, generally from the menstrual cycle, menopause, pregnancy, or, in rare cases, an adrenal or ovarian tumor. Certain drugs, such as progestins (*Provera* and generic), prednisone, and iodine, may also trigger eruptions. If your doctor confirms that it's acne, choose facial cleansers, lotions, or cosmetics that are water-based and oil-free or labeled "noncomedogenic" or "nonacnegenic," meaning that they shouldn't aggravate acne. However, if your face gets flushed or tender when you're breaking out, you may have a relatively common disorder called rosacea. If so, consider keeping a diary to identify what sparks the flare-ups, and try to avoid common triggers, such as stress, alcohol, spicy foods, extreme temperatures, and sun exposure. Prescription tetracycline can often relieve more-severe cases of both rosacea and acne.

TREATING INGROWN TOENAILS

Q *What's the best way to prevent and treat ingrown toenails?*

A Ingrown toenails are generally caused by tight shoes, improperly trimmed nails, or both. Tight shoes can make a corner of the nail curl down and dig into the skin, causing swelling, pain, redness, and even infection. The same problem may develop if you clip the nail short, with no protruding edge at the corner; that invites it to burrow under the skin. To prevent ingrowth, choose shoes that don't crowd the toes, and cut the nails straight across, with the corners extending slightly beyond the end of the toe; gentle filing can eliminate any sharp corners.

To treat an ingrown nail, soak your foot in warm water for 15 to 20 minutes and then tuck a piece of dry cotton under the corner of the nail. Seek professional care if you have a heightened risk of infection, caused by diabetes, poor circulation, or weakened immunity, for example; if you can't reach or manipulate the toe; or if the pain worsens, swelling or drainage develops, or the ingrowth persists. The doctor may prescribe antibiotics or suggest surgical removal of part of the nail.

SKIN SPOTS

Q *I have white spots on the skin of my neck and both hands. I'm embarrassed to be seen in public with this condition, and I've tried skin dyes, but they don't work well. What are these spots, and will anything make them go away?*

A Those spots are the hallmark of vitiligo, a relatively common disorder that destroys pigment cells in the skin. In addition to skin dyes, there are treatments that aim to restore some of the skin's color by stimulating any remaining pigment cells. The usual technique uses topical drugs called psoralens followed by exposure to ultraviolet (UV) light. Unfortunately, that technique works only about half the time and may cause bothersome side effects, such as increased sensitivity to sunlight as well as headaches and nausea.

ANTIWRINKLE WORKOUT?

Q *I've heard that facial exercises are useless for reducing wrinkles. But what about exercises designed to tone the muscles of the neck and lower jaw to prevent or minimize double chin and so-called turkey neck? Are they equally futile?*

A Yes. While a face or jaw workout might tone some muscles, flabby facial muscles aren't a significant cause of sagging skin. The main problem is weakening or damage to the skin itself, caused by heredity, aging, and sun damage. Facial exercises won't counteract the loss of elasticity and fat that leads to skin thinning and drooping. In fact, the repeated stretching involved may even worsen the sagging.

ITCHING ALL OVER

Q *For the past two years, I've itched from my scalp to the soles of my feet, including the palms of my hands, my ears, and my eyes. There is no rash. At night the itching is accompanied by muscular spasms in my legs and a burning sensation.*

A Persistent itching can be caused by allergies to food or medications and by skin disorders such as scabies (which don't always have visible signs). The burning sensation you've experienced could be a sign of nerve inflammation. A physical exam is needed to find the cause of your itching. If your physician can find no treatable cause, he or she may recommend an oral antihistamine to relieve the symptoms.

BAGS UNDER THE EYES

Q *What causes bags under the eyes, and can anything help remove them?*

A As the skin and muscles under the eyes weaken with age, they start to sag and to allow fluid or fat to build up behind them, creating bags. However, many other factors can cause under-eye bags. Temporary ones, for example, could stem from lack of sleep; an allergic reaction to a drug, cosmetic, or environmental irritant; or water retention due to menstruation or pregnancy. Persistent fluid-filled bags can signal a more serious problem, such as thyroid, kidney, liver, or heart disease, all of which can cause water retention. If a physician confirms that tired facial tissue is the culprit, the only means of permanently unpacking the bags is a surgical procedure called blepharoplasty, in which excess skin, muscle, and fat are removed through small incisions.

ROSACEA RX

 Your June 2010 article on rosacea didn't mention laser treatment. Can it help?

 Yes, although it's expensive. Various light therapies can reduce the signs of rosacea, a skin condition that causes facial bumps, flushing, and redness, if simpler measures don't suffice. For example, visible blood vessels on the nose and cheeks can be diminished by pulsed dye lasers, which emit hot yellow light, or by intense pulsed light (IPL), which uses nonlaser light to penetrate the skin. For thickened skin around the nose, doctors might use argon or carbon-dioxide lasers, which can make high-precision surface cuts and can be safer than surgery. But insurance often doesn't cover the cost, about $300 to $600 per treatment, with several sessions typically needed.

CAUSE OF CONSTANT FLUSHING

I'm 85 years old and my face has recently become flushed all the time. What could cause that?

There are a few well-known causes of constant facial flushing: certain daily drugs; a skin condition called rosacea; a handful of rare disorders, including blood, thyroid, and kidney cancers; and a slow-growing tumor called a carcinoid. The most likely drug culprits are cholesterol-cutting niacin and the anti-angina drugs isosorbide (*Isordil, Sorbitrate*, and generic) and nitroglycerin (*Nitro-Dur, Nitrostat*, and generic). Other drugs taken occasionally or briefly may cause temporary flushing; they include the antibiotic rifampin (*Rifadin*), the immunosuppressant cyclosporine (*Sandimmune*), the erectile dysfunction drugs sildenafil (*Viagra*) and vardenafil (*Levitra*), and the steroid triamcinolone (*Aristocort* and generic). Other causes of temporary flushing include alcohol, strong emotions, spicy or bitter foods, the food additives MSG and sodium nitrite, and menopause.

CUCUMBERS AND SKIN

Q *Is it true that putting cucumbers on your skin makes it look smoother?*

A There's no good evidence to support the notion that topical use of cucumbers can improve the texture of your skin or help your complexion in any other way. It's true that cucumbers have a high water content (95 percent!), and adequate hydration is recommended for reducing the appearance of wrinkles. But that refers to water you drink, not apply externally. Putting cucumbers on your skin—for example, over your closed eyes after a long day—might *feel* good, since the temperature inside a cucumber can be up to 20° lower than air temperature and thus provide a cooling effect. Otherwise, save the cukes for eating.

REMOVING BLACKHEADS

Q *What's the safest, most effective way to remove blackheads on the nose or elsewhere on the face?*

A If your blackheads are associated with facial acne, seek professional help because of the possibility of infection. For the occasional blackhead, first wash your face (and hands) with soap and warm water, then, using a blackhead remover, press down the skin around the blackhead to extrude the oxidized matter plugging the pore. Contrary to myth, this practice does no harm.

SCRATCHING AN ITCH

Q *For months I've been suffering from an annoying itch. It starts in one spot, I scratch it, and it turns red and bumpy. Then it disappears and starts up again somewhere else. I've been taking an antihistamine, which helps, but I'm worried. What's wrong with me?*

A The red, bumpy rashes you describe are probably the result of scratching, not the cause of the itch. Unexplained generalized itching, called pruritus, has several possible causes. Older people often itch in the winter because their skin becomes drier. Using water-soluble lubricating oils, bathing less frequently, and running a room humidifier may help. Certain systemic diseases, such as diabetes, liver disease, and some forms of cancer, can also cause itching. These can easily be excluded by appropriate tests. If the cause is unknown, antihistamines may help.

HARRIED BY HIVES

Q *About a week ago I suddenly developed hives—blistery blotches on my skin that seem to appear and disappear within a short time. Why would hives wait until I was 67 years old before appearing? What could be causing them?*

A Hives can show up at any age. Unfortunately, their cause remains a mystery nearly 70 percent of the time. Allergies to food, food additives, medication, or other ingested substances probably account for most cases. If the hives recur frequently, keeping a diary of your food and medication might provide a clue to the specific agent. Cold, heat, and even physical pressure can give some people hives as well. Anxiety and emotional upset are overrated as a cause of hives but can provoke an occasional outbreak. Whatever the cause, antihistamines can relieve the discomfort. Occasionally, temporary use of a prescription steroid medication such as prednisone may be necessary.

✚ *Office* **Visit**

To scratch an itch

THOUGH ITCHING IS A UNIVERSAL HUMAN AFFLICTION, SCIENCE still cannot fully explain the exact mechanism by which we perceive an itch—or why scratching provides such fast relief. What we do know is that several chemicals produced by the body can cause itching, the most notorious being histamine. We also know that, though itching and pain sensations are carried by different nerve fibers, there must be interconnections. Very hot or cold applications, for example, can make an itch stop. And oral painkillers can often help relieve it. A study that scanned brain activity in people with deliberately induced itching found that when they were allowed to scratch, areas of their brains associated with unpleasant sensations, such as itching, became less active, while areas associated with pain became more so.

Itching is a symptom that can signal a near-limitless variety of problems, from trivial to life-threatening. If you have a persistent itch, here's how to proceed.

Starting from scratch

Itching can be generalized or limited to one or more specific locations. If the itch is localized and accompanied by a rash, here are the main culprits to investigate, in approximate order of likelihood:

• **Common insect bites.** Bites from mosquitoes or no-see-ums usually require only a cold compress or steroid cream to ease discomfort. Spider bites can cause blistering and ulceration in addition to itching and might require topical antibiotics. If you're stung by a bee, carefully remove the stinger. Consider seeking medical attention when inflammation and swelling extend well beyond the bite site, since you might require oral antihistamines or corticosteroids.

• **Less common insect-related itching.** Scabies (which is diagnosed with a skin biopsy), head and pubic lice (crabs), bedbug bites (mostly on the torso), and flea bites (usually below the knees of dog owners) all cause severe itching. Each requires a specific eradication technique. Over-the-counter permethrin shampoos generally eliminate head and pubic lice and scabies. Call a professional exterminator to get rid of bedbugs. As for fleas, the remedy is to rid your pet of the critters. (Oddly, one of the most consequential insect bites, that of the deer tick that transmits Lyme disease, rarely causes itching.)

• **Fungal infections.** If your itchy rash looks flat and brownish red and is in a dark, warm, moist spot like your groin, armpits, or feet, you probably have a fungal infection. Over-the-counter fungicidal creams, ointments, and powders are the initial treatment of choice, though stubborn infections might require oral prescription medications.

• **Skin allergy.** The red, blistery, sometimes weepy and intensely itchy condition of contact dermatitis is, as its name indicates, caused by direct contact with an allergen. Common culprits are shampoos, heavy metals (especially nickel) in jewelry, elastic in underwear, liquid detergents, poison ivy, and poison oak. But the cause can be difficult to pin down, since it might be as obscure as a single ingredient in a hair spray. Steroid creams can provide some relief until you find and banish the culprit.

Itching all over

With or without a rash, itches that have spread over your whole body sometimes indicate more serious conditions. Common causes include:

• **Dry skin.** This is the most common cause of total body itching and is especially likely in the dehydrated air of heated winter interiors. The main danger of such itching is scratching, which can lead to skin infections caused by resistant bacteria. Faithful use of emollient creams can help, especially after bathing or showering.

• **Hives.** Also known as urticaria, this itchy, generalized rash of red skin bumps or wheals is usually caused by a reaction to medications or foods. Penicillin is a common offender among drugs, and shellfish among foods. If you can identify the cause, stay away from it for good, because it might cause an even more severe reaction the next time. But sometimes the source is never found, in which case you have idiopathic urticaria. Antihistamines and corticosteroids are often necessary.

• **Systemic illnesses.** More rarely, generalized itching, usually without a rash, can signal conditions that include anemia or thyroid, liver, or kidney disease. And at times it can be a tip-off to lymphoma or an underlying internal cancer. If you experience prolonged itching over your whole body that you cannot attribute to an allergic reaction or dry skin, a visit to your doctor is in order.

Stomach ailments

COMBATING CONSTIPATION

Q Can exercise ease constipation?

A Yes—and being inactive can worsen it. Getting 20 to 30 minutes of aerobic activity a day—say, walking—can make it easier to pass stools by speeding up digestion. If you have limited mobility, doing light exercises for the legs and abdomen might also help. If exercise, drinking more fluids, and eating more fiber don't improve symptoms, talk with your doctor, who might order tests to see if you have an intestinal problem or a condition that could contribute to constipation, such as irritable bowel syndrome or a neurologic or endocrine disorder. Biofeedback and pelvic-floor (Kegel) exercises can improve bowel movements if constipation stems from inadequate muscle tone in the rectum.

GASTRITIS RELIEF

Q I often have upper-abdominal pain stemming from gastritis. What causes that?

A Anything that inflames the stomach lining can spark gastritis, a sometimes sharp but often dull, gnawing upper abdominal pain that can be accompanied by belching, bloating, and nausea. Heartburn may cause similar symptoms, but that pain typically is a burning sensation in the center of the chest, behind the breastbone. The three most common causes of stomach-lining inflammation are:
 • Increased secretion of stomach acid, stimulated by coffee, tea, alcohol, or cigarettes.

• Direct irritation by a food such as hot peppers or by a medication, particularly a nonsteroidal anti-inflammatory drug (NSAID) such as aspirin, ibuprofen (*Advil* and generic), or naproxen (*Aleve* and generic).

• Erosion of the stomach's mucus barrier, most often caused by prolonged use of NSAIDs.

You may be able to pacify the pain by avoiding those provoking substances and taking nonprescription heartburn drugs such as famotidine (*Pepcid AC* and generic) or ranitidine (*Zantac 150* and generic). If those measures fail, your doctor may prescribe a more potent acid-reducer such as lansoprazole (*Prevacid, Prevacid 24HR*, and generic) or omeprazole (*Prilosec, Prilosec OTC*, and generic).

ARTIFICIAL SUGAR AND BELLY PAIN

Q *After eating sugar-free jelly beans, my husband developed severe stomach cramps. Is there anything in sugar-free foods that could cause that problem?*

A Yes. Such foods are often sweetened with substances called sugar alcohols, which can cause stomach cramps and diarrhea. Those sweeteners appear on labels with such names as erythritol, lactitol, maltitol, mannitol, sorbitol, and xylitol. If you're sensitive to sugar alcohols, as little as 10 to 15 grams—the typical amount in one to two servings of sweetened food—can trigger gastrointestinal distress.

WHEN TO TEST YOUR GUT FOR BUGS

Q *For several years I suffered from an ulcer. But it wasn't until I was tested for H. pylori, the Helicobacter pylori bacterium, that my doctor discovered I had an infection and* *needed antibiotics. When should people get tested for this bug?*

A Since *H. pylori* is quite common but usually harmless—causing ulcers, in up to 10 percent of infected people, and possibly contributing to stomach cancer in a much smaller fraction—testing is generally warranted in only two circumstances: if you have ulcers that can't be explained by the most common cause, regularly taking nonsteroidal anti-inflammatory drugs like aspirin or ibuprofen (*Advil, Motrin,* and generic), or if you have a close family history of stomach cancer. (Symptoms of ulcers include a dull, gnawing ache below the breast bone that typically eases during meals, worsens one to three hours later, and intensifies during the night.)

Killing *H. pylori* usually requires a combination of certain antibiotics and an acid reducer such as lansoprazole (*Prevacid, Prevacid 24HR,* and generic) or omeprazole (*Prilosec, Prilosec OTC,* and generic). If those medications fail, a more invasive examination of the stomach and upper intestine may be required to rule out other conditions, followed by a different combination of antibiotics.

SOY AND HEARTBURN

Q *I quit drinking dairy milk because I learned that it can trigger my heartburn. Is soy milk a good alternative?*

A Possibly, if your symptoms really are caused or worsened by dairy foods, and if soy doesn't cause the same problems. But be wary of what you pair with your soy milk, since caffeinated drinks like coffee and tea can themselves trigger heartburn. And some people experience other gastrointestinal problems from soy, such as bloating, diarrhea, and flatulence. But if you can tolerate it, there are good reasons to make the switch. Two to three daily servings of soy protein might help lower LDL (bad) cholesterol.

And most soy milk is fortified with calcium and vitamin D, which can help replace what you're not getting from dairy products.

FLATULENCE

Q *I've recently begun suffering from flatulence. I'm 65 and have no obvious digestive problems. What could be causing this often embarrassing problem?*

A It could be the food you eat. Intestinal gas is the price some people pay for good nutrition. Intestinal bacteria can ferment the remnants of certain carbohydrates, thereby producing gas. Likely culprits include bran and whole grains, as well as many fruits and vegetables, such as apples, avocados, beans, broccoli, cabbage, cauliflower, corn, cucumbers, melons, onions, peas, peppers, and radishes. Sometimes milk and other lactose-containing products (ice cream, puddings, custards) are at fault. Try cutting out suspect foods for a while, and see if it helps.

Swallowed air can also produce a small amount of gas. It may help to eat more slowly, chew with your mouth closed, and avoid gulping food. Over-the-counter remedies such as simethicone (*Gas-X, Mylanta Gas Relief,* and generic) and charcoal tablets are not usually very helpful. Flatulence is nothing to worry about unless it's accompanied by a recent change in bowel habits such as constipation or diarrhea. That could indicate an underlying disorder such as an intestinal infection or tumor, irritable bowel syndrome (spastic colon), or poor food absorption.

✚ *Office* **Visit**

Intestinal gas: A right of passage?

"MAY I PLEASE CLOSE THE DOOR?" THE SLIGHT, 58-YEAR-OLD school librarian asked in hushed tones. Leaning forward, she confided the reason for her visit. Her inability to control the passage of odoriferous gas, she said, was causing her severe anxiety and rendering her an outcast on the job. "They have me working in the stacks two days a week now," she said. Whether her assumption of cause and effect was real or not, the matter was obviously a source of great concern to her. Every living creature who possesses a digestive tract passes gas each and every day. For humans it starts as soon as we're born and ends a day or so after we die. Despite the universality of this physiologic process, the passage of gas is considered the basest of bodily functions, often assigned to the most ill-mannered of individuals, as in the writings of Chaucer and Shakespeare, or used as a sound gag at a party (whoopee cushions have been around for hundreds of years).

How flatulence happens

The average person produces one to three pints of gas per day and eliminates it in 14 to 23 passes, some while asleep. More than 99 percent of this gas mixture is odorless, and consists of carbon dioxide, nitrogen, and oxygen, which we inadvertently swallow when we eat, drink carbonated beverages, chew gum, or smoke. Some carbon dioxide is made in the stomach.

In addition, the normal bacterial population of our colon (large bowel) produces a tiny amount of hydrogen gas and methane by fermenting the carbohydrates left over from the small intestinal digestive process and forming hydrogen sulfide (like the smell of rotten eggs), methanethiol (like the smell of decomposing vegetables), and dimethyl sulfide (a heavy sweetish odor). In fact, less than 1 percent of the gas we produce accounts for all of the odor.

Passing that gas mixture causes the anal sphincter to vibrate, producing a veritable symphony of sounds depending on the force with which the gas is expelled and the resistance of the sphincter. Who can forget that rousing campfire scene from Mel Brooks's 1974 masterpiece, *Blazing Saddles*?

When excess gas occurs alongside nausea, vomiting, diarrhea, constipation, or involuntary weight loss, the need to see a physician is obvious. But by and large, gas as an isolated complaint is rarely due to a serious disorder. When a patient comes to me complaining about excess gas, a careful history, a physical exam, and a few well-chosen laboratory tests can rule out those few, more notable, causes: irritable bowel syndrome, lactose intolerance, celiac disease, or gastroesophageal reflux disorder. In the vast majority of cases, flatulence indicates nothing more than that the patient is alive and eating a healthy diet.

Gas reduction

To reduce smelly gas production, the traditional approach is to cut down on foods that produce high residues of indigestible carbohydrates. These include:

• Corn, noodles, and potatoes, and most foods high in dietary fiber.

• Fructose, found in artichokes, onions, pears, and wheat.

• Raffinose, found in asparagus, beans, broccoli, brussels sprouts, cabbage, and whole grains.

• Sorbitol, found in apples, peaches, pears, prunes, and candies and drinks that use it as a sweetener.

Only those items that seem to be the largest contributors need to be eliminated. One commercial over-the-counter product, *Beano*, may reduce the amount of gas formed from foods containing raffinose.

As for the incriminating and distinctive sound, patients can try to reduce the magnitude of the expulsive force, use the holdback technique, or try more opportune timing.

To mask odor, bismuth subsalicylate (*Pepto-Bismol* and generic) can be helpful in reducing the smell of hydrogen sulfide gas but probably should not be taken on a long-term basis because of possible toxicity. Chlorophyll tablets are usually a waste of time. Simethicone (*Gas-X*, *Mylicon*, and generic) makes small bubbles into larger ones and may help with belching but does little for lower intestinal gas. Using activated charcoal to soak up the gas is another possibility, although the amount that is needed by mouth is too large to be practical. A better solution is activated charcoal-coated underwear or pads worn inside underwear.

Our librarian managed to cut back on her raffinose containing carbohydrates. She also wears an activated charcoal pad and has trained herself to pass gas more quietly. And she is no longer ridden with anxiety since finding out that everyone takes a turn at working the stacks.

✚ Office Visit

When the going gets tough

REMEMBER SUMMER CAMP? CAREFREE DAYS OF NEW friendships, arts and crafts, swimming and boating, noisy mess halls, sing-along campfires, and the quiet time at the end of the day, followed by "Taps" and lights out. But not before the camp nurse, in her starched white uniform, made her appearance, clipboard and pencil in hand, and directed the question of the day to each, in turn: "Soft, medium, hard, or none?"—and she wasn't taking egg orders for breakfast. A teaspoon of castor oil was the unwary respondent's reward.

Although that barbaric ritual has gone the way of public hangings, America's obsession with daily bowel movements has persisted, largely due to persistent misconceptions. One myth is that waste products can accumulate and contaminate the rest of the body. Another is the belief that constipation can cause colon cancer.

Patients have varying ideas about what constitutes constipation. One survey of nearly 600 constipated patients found that the main complaint of 79 percent was straining to pass the stool. Hard stools were a problem for 71 percent, while 57 percent complained of infrequent bowel movements. (Some had more than one complaint.)

The standard medical definition of constipation includes both of the following: 1. infrequency (less than three bowel movements per week); and 2. difficult passage of hard, dry stools. Most everyone agrees that anything between three times a week to three times a day can be considered normal.

Constipation, as defined above, affects as many as one of every four Americans at one time or another, occurs more than twice as often in women as in men, and is more frequent among older people.

The cause may vary

Most of the time constipation is transient and related to changes in diet or schedule. Going on vacation, starting the Atkins diet, cutting out your usual exercise routine, or ignoring the morning urge in order to catch a train can play havoc with your bowels. A host of medications can cause constipation, including iron and calcium supplements, antidepressants, painkillers, and some blood-pressure drugs.

Constipation can occur in pregnancy or be caused by serious conditions, such as an underactive thyroid, elevated blood-calcium levels, Parkinson's disease, multiple sclerosis, irritable bowel syndrome, and actual blockages of the intestine by colon cancer. All can cause difficulty in moving one's bowels.

Loosening up

Although a lack of fiber in the diet and dehydration can cause constipation, treating the problem by increasing dietary fiber and drinking eight glasses of water a day lacks the certainty of evidence-based medicine and often results in bloating, flatulence, abdominal distention, and increased urinary frequency. As long as you're consuming adequate amounts of fiber (at least 25 grams per day) and drinking enough fluids to keep your urine a pale yellow, increases are not likely to help.

Resuming your usual lifestyle after a vacation or switching the medication that was the cause usually does the trick. You won't suffer permanent harm from a few days of constipation, but there's nothing wrong with the temporary use of a laxative if you're truly uncomfortable. But how to choose from the myriad products that line the shelves of your pharmacy?

The trick is to select a single-ingredient product that matches your particular complaint. If your main symptom is straining to pass hard, dry stools, try polyethylene glycol (*Miralax* and generic) or consider docusate *(Colace* and generic), an emollient type of laxative better known as a stool softener. If your problem is infrequency, choose a bulk laxative such as methylcellulose *(Citrucel* and generic), polycarbophil *(Equalactin, FiberCon,* and generic), or psyllium *(Fiberall, Metamucil,* and generic). If you have both complaints, take both kinds. Despite lore to the contrary, both types of laxatives are relatively safe for long-term use, but check with your physician.

For more stubborn cases, as can occur in seniors with aging bowels, the occasional use of a stimulant laxative such as bisacodyl *(Correctol, Dulcolax,* and generic) may be necessary. Drawbacks are painful cramping and diarrhea with urgency. As with any symptom treated with an over-the-counter medication, if constipation persists longer than a week or two or recurs after treatment, it's time to see your physician to find out if something more serious is going on.

The thyroid

THYROID-PILL DEPENDENCY?

Q I've taken a small dose of thyroid hormone every day for 40 years. My doctor hadn't diagnosed hypothyroidism; he just recommended the medication for chronic fatigue. Should I stop taking it?

A Probably. However, even though you may not have really needed the drug initially, your thyroid gland has adjusted to the supplement by decreasing its normal production of thyroid hormone. So if you go off the drug now, your thyroid gland could take up to six weeks to recover and you might suffer temporary symptoms of hypothyroidism, such as weight gain and sluggishness. Still, it's better to avoid medication when your body can do the job itself. If you're willing to put up with those symptoms for a few weeks, talk to your physician about discontinuing the pills.

UNDERACTIVE THYROID?

Q According to a popular medical book, I may have an underactive thyroid gland. My hair, skin, eyes, and mouth are very dry; I have puffiness under my eyes, and I'm very sensitive to cold on my back. But a blood test indicates my thyroid is normal. Are there other ways I should be tested for an underactive thyroid?

A Not if you've had the two appropriate blood tests. One measures thyroid hormone itself, and one measures thyroid-stimulating hormone, or TSH. Your symptoms could be caused by many other problems, including dry environment, medical conditions that dry out the eyes, and certain skin diseases.

+ *Office* **Visit**

The dangers of silent thyroid disease

A FEW MONTHS AGO I SAW TWO WOMEN, BACK-TO-BACK, WHO were practically diagnostic mirror images. Each was referred by a colleague puzzled by the results of routine thyroid-function tests. Neither had complaints that could be considered thyroid-related. Both had perfectly normal blood levels of the two thyroid hormones (T3 and T4) but abnormal levels on a third test of thyroid function called thyroid stimulating hormone (TSH). One woman's TSH was low and the other's was elevated. Should both be treated? One? And, if so—which one?

Before going any further, let me explain how the normal thyroid works. (Bear with me; it's complicated.)

The butterfly-shaped thyroid gland sits just below the Adam's apple. It takes orders from the pituitary gland—the peanut-sized master endocrine gland situated below the base of the brain. Those orders take the form of TSH, a hormone that tells the thyroid gland to make T4, a pro-hormone, which is converted in the liver to an active hormone, T3. The latter then enters the cells of the body, where it does its job: stimulating metabolism. Without T3 and T4, we would slowly wind down like an old-fashioned record player; with too much our metabolism races out of control. But T3 and T4 also play a feedback role in the regulation of pituitary TSH production. When levels of T3 and T4 increase, signaling a sufficient supply, TSH levels go down, and vice versa. What can make it confusing is that even when T3 and T4 are in the normal range, minor fluctuations can cause significant changes in TSH blood levels.

Subclinical disease

Two conditions, neither of which produce clinical symptoms (that's why they're called subclinical), are both characterized by normal T3 and T4 levels. But one (subclinical hyperthyroidism) features low TSH levels and the other (subclinical hypothyroidism) is characterized by elevated TSH levels. Those two disorders were unknown before sensitive TSH assays became available.

At first we endocrinologists thought we could ignore what was considered "pre-disease," or at best follow it intermittently, until and unless symptomatic hyperthyroidism or hypothyroidism developed. But while transitions to overt disease were few and far between, evidence has emerged suggesting that the subclinical conditions may not be so benign after all.

A recent analysis in the *Archives of Internal Medicine* concluded that subclinical hyperthyroidism (normal T3 and T4, low TSH), which affects about 1 percent of adults, was associated not only with increased mortality but also with heart disease—specifically, atrial fibrillation. And the lower the TSH, the higher the risk of complications. Other researchers have found increased evidence of osteoporosis, especially in older women, which improved following the institution of anti-thyroid treatment.

Subclinical hypothyroidism seems to be a more common but less dire problem. It occurs in perhaps 10 percent of the population. The most common cause is autoimmune thyroiditis, also known as Hashimoto's disease, in which a person's immune system attacks his or her own thyroid. About one in five cases will progress to full-fledged hypothyroidism. Some studies have suggested a link to heart disease secondary to the elevated cholesterol levels seen in many people with subclinical hypothyroidism. But treatment remains controversial when TSH levels are less than 10mIU/ml. The higher the TSH, the more certain are the benefits of treatment.

Whom to treat

The first patient (the one with subclinical hyperthyroidism) was a 75-year-old retired schoolteacher with diabetes, moderate osteoporosis, and a history of hypertension. In view of her bone disease and cardiovascular risk, I treated her with methimazole (*Tapazole* and generic), a medication that blocks the synthesis of T4. Within several weeks, her TSH ascended into normal range. She has tolerated the medication well. The second patient (the one with subclinical hypothyroidism) was a 48-year-old yoga instructor in good health. Her TSH was 7mIU/ml and thyroid autoantibodies were not detected. We decided to do nothing. I am following her periodically with TSH measurements. If her TSH climbs and she develops symptoms, we will discuss treatment with thyroid hormone.

GOITERS AND DIET

Q *I've read that soybeans contain substances that can interfere with thyroid hormones, possibly causing goiters. I like soy milk and tofu, but I'm concerned because I take the thyroid hormone levothyroxine* (Synthroid) *to treat an underactive thyroid gland. Should I stop eating soy foods?*

A No—but you should be careful about when you eat it. Soybeans and certain vegetables such as cabbage, cassava, rutabagas, and turnips contain substances called goitrogens, which tend to inhibit production of thyroid hormones. But the amount of goitrogens in those foods is so small that even with an underactive thyroid, you'd have to eat shovelsful before they caused even a mild problem, let alone goiters, or visibly enlarged thyroid glands. However, soy may interfere with thyroid hormones in a different way: It appears to inhibit the body's absorption of the hormone pills. So you should probably consume soy at least eight hours before or after you take the levothyroxine.

Vaccines

ADULT IMMUNIZATIONS

Q *How often do adults need to have a tetanus shot?*

A All adults should receive a tetanus-diphtheria toxoid booster every 10 years. If an injury that might lead to tetanus occurs more than five years after the last shot, another booster should be given. (The next shot would then be given 10 years from that date.)

FLU SHOTS

Q *I've heard so many opinions, pro and con, about flu shots. Who should get a flu shot? How effective is it? When is the best time to get one?*

A Anyone who can tolerate a flu shot should consider getting one before the influenza season begins. That's especially important for these high-risk groups:
- Children age 6 months to 18 years.
- People age 50 or over.
- People with chronic lung or heart disorders, including children with asthma.
- Adults and children who, during the preceding year, needed regular medical care or hospitalization for a chronic disease: diabetes, kidney disorders, sickle-cell disease, or suppressed immune systems (including HIV/AIDS).
- Children and teenagers 6 months to 18 years who are on long-term aspirin therapy.

• People who live with or care for a person at high risk. A flu shot takes about two weeks to provide protection and lasts about six months. But the injection does not provide full immunity in all cases. The shot generally prevents the flu in about 60 percent of healthy people in their sixties, though that varies on just how well the vaccine developed that year matches the virus that actually emerges. Younger adults and children typically benefit even more from the shots. If an unexpected strain of flu pops up during the flu season, the vaccine may not work at all.

Generally, October is the best time for a flu shot, but anytime between September and February is better than not at all. Travelers abroad, however, should consider a flu shot whatever the month. They may risk exposure to the virus at any time of year.

PERTUSSIS AND MEDICARE

Q *Does Medicare cover the pertussis vaccine?*

A It depends on the plan. The tetanus-diphtheria-acellular pertussis vaccine, or Tdap, prevents whooping cough (pertussis), a highly contagious bacterial infection that can last for weeks or months and in rare cases can be fatal. Tdap previously wasn't recommended for people 65 and older, but the federal government's Advisory Committee on Immunization Practices now recommends that all adults receive the vaccine, regardless of when they had their last plain tetanus shot. It isn't covered under Original Medicare or Medicare Part A but is covered under the optional Medicare Part D prescription-drug program, though you may still have a co-payment. Without insurance, the shot usually costs $60 to $100.

JUST ONE SHOT FOR PNEUMONIA?

Q *You've said that people 65 and older should receive pneumococcal vaccine just once. But some doctors have told me they recommend the shot every five years. I had one six years ago when I was 71. Should I get another?*

A Healthy older people generally need only one dose of pneumococcal vaccine. (However, a single revaccination with the "23-valent" vaccine is worth considering if you previously received the older, "14-valent" type of pneumococcal vaccine.) But if you have a medical condition such as heart, kidney, liver, or lung disease, diabetes, Hodgkin's disease, cerebrospinal fluid leaks, an immune-system disorder, or sickle-cell anemia, you could be susceptible to complications from pneumonia. Anyone in those risk groups should get a shot every six years.

PERTUSSIS SHOT

Q Who should get the pertussis vaccine?

A There are several vaccines that are used to prevent pertussis. In the U.S., the DTaP vaccine is given to children under age 7 and two vaccines (the Tdap and Td) are given to older children and adults. The vaccine, called Tdap, is recommended as a single shot for anyone age 11 and older, either by itself or in place of one Td (tetanus and diphtheria) booster. Pertussis, or whooping cough, is a highly infectious bacterial illness that causes violent coughing followed by a loud, gasping "whoop." While a previous case might offer some temporary immunity, the effect wanes over time. Tell the provider if you've experienced severe allergic reactions previously.

SHINGLES VACCINE

Q *I'm 77 and recently had shingles. Should I still get the vaccine?*

A It's not a bad idea. The vaccine reduces not only the risk of getting shingles—a painful, blistering rash caused by the reactivation of the virus that causes chicken pox—but the severity of the illness if you do get it. That's an important benefit, since shingles can cause nerve pain that lasts for months or even years, and in rare cases can lead to vision or hearing loss, infections, and pneumonia. While getting shingles twice isn't common, it does occur, so it makes sense to do what you can to prevent or lessen a repeat case. Make sure the rash is completely gone before getting the shot, and tell the doctor providing it that you recently had shingles.

SHINGLES AND STROKE

Q *Does a recent case of shingles increase a person's stroke risk?*

A Yes, by about 30 percent in the year following the shingles, according to a recent study published in the journal *Stroke*. It's not clear whether shingles caused most of the strokes or if underlying factors put the patients at heightened risk for both shingles and stroke. It does appear that people are more likely to have a stroke if their shingles affected the nerves around the eye (herpes zoster opthalmicus). And severe cases of any form of shingles can spread to the spinal cord or brain, which could trigger a stroke. That's all the more reason to get the shingles vaccine *(Zostavax)*, particularly if you're between 60 and 69, the group for which it's most effective.

✚ *Office* Visit

Why we need vaccines

THE SUMMER OF 1949 STANDS OUT IN MY MEMORY AS THE time my younger brother nearly died. He was 16 and a junior counselor at a children's summer camp in Connecticut. Midway through the season, a few campers came down with sore throats and fever. And soon, a few counselors took sick as well. Jack was one of them. It wasn't long before the infirmary overflowed, the camp was closed, and everyone was sent home. Jack was told he had bulbar poliomyelitis and was admitted to the contagious disease section of the local county hospital. Fortunately his respiratory muscles were not affected. After a few weeks he began to recover and eventually was discharged with intact muscle function. Four of the kids from his camp were not so lucky; they died.

And that was only the beginning of the epidemic. Three years later, the number of polio cases reached nearly 60,000, making it one of the worst epidemics in U.S. history. More than 3,000 people died and more than 21,000 were left with mild to disabling paralysis.

A history lesson

In early April 1955, as an intern attending a scientific meeting in Atlantic City, N.J., I heard Jonas Salk describe the results of a preliminary study demonstrating the efficacy of his polio vaccine. The thunderous applause lasted at least 10 minutes. Shortly afterward, on April 12, 10 years to the day after the death of President Franklin D. Roosevelt (himself a polio survivor), a much-anticipated radio broadcast proclaimed Salk's vaccine safe and effective. As its use became widespread, the number of polio cases quickly began to dwindle, and it has now been eliminated in this country. The last reported case originating in the Western Hemisphere was in Peru in 1991.

Of all the advances in medicine during the course of the last century or two—including anesthesia, antibiotics, sterile surgical techniques, cancer chemotherapy, and the prevention of heart attacks and strokes—probably none has had a greater impact on human sickness and death than the widespread use of vaccines. Smallpox, a scourge that killed millions through the centuries, is now a distant memory; the world's last case was in 1977 in Somalia. Vaccines have significantly reduced the number of reported cases of disease. Diphtheria and invasive hemophilus influenzae B have been cut by 100 percent; mumps, by 96 percent; tetanus, 93 percent; whooping cough, 92 percent; hepatitis A, 87 percent; chicken pox, 85 percent; and acute hepatitis B, 80 percent. The decline in cases of pneumococcal pneumonia has been only 34 percent, probably because many of the elderly or chronically ill adults who need the vaccine don't get it.

Get your shots

Despite the formidable weight of evidence that vaccines prevent or reduce the severity of many infectious diseases, a substantial but vocal minority of people not only refuse vaccinations for themselves and their children but also advocate against the use of vaccines by others. The reasons vary but basically hinge on the belief that vaccines are harmful. At one point or another, anti-vaccinationists have blamed vaccines for attention deficit hyperactivity disorder, autism, brain damage, and multiple sclerosis.

Many well-designed scientific studies have found that such blame is misplaced. Reactions in the first days after a vaccination can include a sore arm, fever, aches, and pains, but these are minor, usually well-tolerated, and resolve quickly. A more serious reaction can occur, usually after four or more weeks, but it's rare. For example, the risk of brain inflammation after a measles vaccination is one in a million. But the risk after natural infection with the measles virus is much greater—one in 1,000 cases. The estimated incidence of Guillain-Barré syndrome, a serious paralytic neurological disorder, after influenza vaccination is about one in a million, but its natural incidence in the population at large is even greater—10 to 20 cases per million adults.

In the U.S. we now have immunization guidelines for 17 vaccine-preventable diseases. Benefits for all those vaccines far outweigh any risks. During your next office visit, make a point to ask your doctor what, if any, shots or boosters you need (not all vaccine protection lasts forever), especially against tetanus, diphtheria, and whooping cough; pneumonia; hepatitis A and B; shingles; and the human papilloma virus.

Vitamins and supplements

VITAMINS AND THE FLU

Q *Can taking vitamins help prevent the flu?*

A Probably not. It's true that an adequate intake of vitamins A, C, D, E, and the B vitamins, as well as iron, zinc, and healthful probiotic bacteria, help to maintain a strong immune system, which improves your ability to fight off illness. But there's no solid clinical-trial evidence that supplements of vitamins offer additional protection against the flu.

MAD-COW SUPPLEMENTS?

Q *You reported that some dietary supplements contain the animal parts most likely to harbor the mutant protein that causes mad-cow disease. How can I spot those supplements?*

A Check the ingredients label. Any animal tissue in a supplement should be clearly listed there. The most infectious tissues come from the central-nervous and lymphatic systems—including the brain, heart, liver, lungs, spleen, and thymus—as well as from the intestines. They're usually found in glandular supplements, which contain organ extracts from animals that purportedly boost the function of the corresponding human organs. While the risk of contracting mad-cow disease from such supplements is currently very small, you might still want to avoid them, particularly since the evidence of any benefit is tenuous at best.

SILVER SUPPLEMENTS

Q *Are there any benefits to taking colloidal silver supplements?*

A No—and silver can be hazardous. The supplements, which contain tiny silver particles suspended in liquid, have been touted as a nutritional supplement for pregnant women and a treatment for allergies, arthritis, cancer, diabetes, and infection. But silver provides no known nutritional benefits. While some evidence suggests it may have mild germ-killing powers, it's too weak and too toxic to be used as an antibiotic. And there's no other plausible explanation for how it might fight disease or protect either the fetus or the mother; in fact, increased blood levels of silver during pregnancy have been linked to birth defects. While decades of consuming trace amounts of the mineral found in some foods and drinking water contribute to such elevated levels, supplements are a more likely cause. Possible toxic effects, in addition to birth defects, include a permanent bluish discoloration of the fingernails, gums, skin, and whites of the eyes and, in more severe cases, organ damage and neurologic disorders. In theory, silver may also interfere with certain antibiotics as well as with drugs for hypertension or thyroid disease.

✚ Office Visit

Vitamin B12: Panacea or placebo?

"HEY, DOC, I'VE BEEN DRAGGING LATELY. HOW ABOUT A SHOT of B12? My mother-in-law had one, and it put her on top of the world."

Primary-care practitioners have been fielding such requests about this reputedly potent fatigue-fighter for at least a half-century. So you would think the revitalizing properties of B12 for healthy individuals would be well established by now. Well, think again. And you might also be surprised by how many people truly are B12 deficient.

The oversized reputation of B12 probably stems from long-ago research at Boston City Hospital that established the vitamin's importance in relieving the fatigue associated with pernicious anemia, a disease that impairs the absorption of B12 from food.

The injectable red liquid quickly gained a reputation as a magic antidote for everyday fatigue in otherwise healthy people with normal vitamin B12 blood levels. This belief has persisted despite the lack of good scientific evidence for its use as an all-purpose energizer. In 1985 a National Ambulatory Medical Care Survey recorded about 2.5 million B12 injections, of which fewer than 400,000 were for diagnoses compatible with B12-deficiency disorders.

When to treat

It wasn't until 1973 that the first randomized controlled clinical trial—involving 29 subjects and lasting only six weeks—took place. The participants, all with normal vitamin B12 blood levels, were given either a twice-weekly dose of the vitamin or a placebo for two weeks, followed by a rest period of two weeks, and a final two-week phase in which the vitamin and placebo recipients were secretly switched. The study was flawed because only the group that received the vitamin first was analyzed. No statistical differences were noted in appetite, sleep patterns, and fatigue, but those initially given B12 were "happier" and "felt better."

In another small randomized controlled study from 1989, 15 people with chronic fatigue syndrome were given a mixture of liver extract, folic acid, and B12, or a placebo, at different phases of the month-long study. Their fatigue levels were the same regardless of which phase they were in.

The role of vitamin B12 has been much better established as replacement therapy for people who are really deficient in the vitamin, which is essential for DNA synthesis, red blood cell development, peripheral nerve integrity, and cognitive function. B12 is not made in our bodies and can be obtained only from animal proteins (or artificially fortified grains). Once it's ingested, stomach acid is necessary to pry it from food, after which the vitamin combines with something called intrinsic factor, a substance made in the stomach, before eventually being absorbed in the small intestine.

Whom to test

According to the 2001-2004 National Health and Nutrition Examination Survey, 3.2 percent of those over the age of 50 have true B12 deficiency. More in that age group are at risk; up to 30 percent lack sufficient stomach acid to extract B12 from food. Even greater decreases in stomach acid can occur in patients using proton pump inhibitors, such as omeprazole (*Prilosec* and generic) and esomeprazole (*Nexium*); and H2 blockers, such as famotidine (*Pepcid* and generic) and ranitidine (*Zantac* and generic). Another medication associated with B12 deficiency is the diabetes drug metformin (*Glucophage* and generic). Strict vegetarians should consume extra B12 from either fortified food or supplements. Malabsorption due to inflammatory bowel disease (Crohn's and regional ileitis) can also cause a deficiency.

There are no current guidelines on screening for B12 deficiency in people without symptoms. Still, it seems reasonable to check high-risk individuals, especially since oral vitamin B12 has now been shown to be as effective as injected B12, and in any event, supplementation is not harmful.

Ask your physician to check your vitamin B12 level if you:

• are over 50 years old
• take a PPI or an H2 blocker
• take metformin
• are a strict vegetarian
• have inflammatory bowel disease.

FAT-SOLUBLE VITAMINS

Q *You've reported that some fat in the stomach is necessary in order to absorb vitamin D from food. Does it matter what type of fat?*

A Not in terms of absorption, but you should stick mainly to unsaturated fats, found in fish and most vegetable oils, rather than saturated ones, which can raise LDL (bad) cholesterol. Foods that contain those healthful fats are themselves often rich in fat-soluble vitamins, which include A, E, and K in addition to D. Good sources include avocados, nuts, vegetable oils, and fatty fish such as wild salmon and trout. But don't take the need for a little fat as license to overdo it. Even when it's the healthful kind, fat should account for only about 15 to 35 percent of your daily calories.

VITAMIN D AND WINDOW LIGHT

Q *Recently, you reported that people generally need some sun exposure to maintain adequate vitamin D levels. But does sunlight passing through windows trigger production of vitamin D?*

A No. Glass blocks ultraviolet B (UVB) radiation, the type that stimulates vitamin D synthesis by the skin. To get enough of the vitamin, you probably need to briefly expose some skin to direct sunlight a few days a week during the warmer months— unless you take a multivitamin containing D or consume lots of D-fortified milk plus some fatty fish. However, you can get sunburned through a window. That's because windows don't block UVA, the other harmful type of radiation from sunlight, unless the glass is specially coated or tinted. Like UVB, UVA can cause sunburn and skin aging as well as an increased risk of skin cancer and possibly cataracts and macular degeneration. So apply sunscreen if you're driving or just sitting in front of a window in bright sunlight for more than about 20 minutes in most parts of North America, and less than that in southern states in the U.S.

✚ *Office***Visit**

The perils of dietary supplements

A 74-YEAR-OLD LICENSED PRACTICAL NURSE CAME TO THE emergency room with a dangerously high blood pressure of 200/120. Emergency measures averted the risk of a stroke or heart attack and reduced her pressure to acceptable levels. One month previously, she had stopped taking her prescription blood-pressure medicine in favor of hawthorn and forskolin, herbal supplements she found on the Internet.

A 23-year-old graduate student with a history of multiple respiratory allergies including ragweed was seen in the office after four days of increasingly severe asthma and trouble breathing. He was admitted to a hospital and required a prednisone treatment to break the attack. He recalled that a week before he had felt a cold coming on and, not wanting to miss classes, took several tablets of echinacea, a botanical supplement, supplied by a friend.

A 75-year-old attorney with chronic atrial fibrillation came in for his monthly clotting-time test, necessary because he was on medication to prevent stroke-causing clots from forming in his heart. The test indicated a dangerously high risk of bleeding, and he was hospitalized while his dose was carefully adjusted. He admitted that for the past month he had been taking large doses of ginkgo biloba on the advice of a client who swore the herb would prevent dementia.

An unregulated industry

The late Edward H. Rynearson, M.D., a professor of medicine at the Mayo Clinic, said it all in a 1974 article in the journal *Nutrition Reviews* titled "Americans Love Hogwash." He wrote that the most widespread quackery in the U.S. was the promotion of vitamins and dietary supplements. Today the industry has grown into a more than $28 billion-a-year behemoth. More than half of Americans use dietary supplements despite the fact that none of them are required to be screened for efficacy or safety.

In the early 1990s, the Food and Drug Administration, concerned by reports of adverse reactions caused by widespread supplement use, began to crack down on the burgeoning industry. A lobbying campaign by supplement makers and marketers led to the passage of the Dietary Supplement Health and Education Act in 1994 by a misguided Congress in the belief that it was protecting a consumer's right to choose among health-care options. In effect, the law prevents the FDA from interfering with the marketing of any product defined as a dietary supplement—including vitamins, minerals, herbals, botanicals, and amino acids. All regulatory barriers effectively swept aside, the industry exploded to the point that today some 55,000 products are on the market, compared with just 4,000 in 1994. If the FDA wants to remove a supplement from the market, the law requires the agency to follow a burdensome process to prove the product is unsafe. Consequently, in all these years the agency has managed to ban only one ingredient, ephedra. Until 2007 the government didn't even require manufacturers to report serious adverse events to the FDA.

How to protect yourself

Ignore or view with extreme skepticism the claims in dietary supplement ads, especially the ones that turn up when you use a Web search engine. Here are some other tips:

• Instead of listening to well-meaning friends or even your own spouse or partner, research supplements and other health matters on trustworthy sites such as ConsumerReports.org, FDA.gov, MedlinePlus.gov, and USP.org.

• Don't mistake "natural" for safe. A growing list of "natural" dietary supplements has been linked to kidney problems, liver disease, nerve damage, and even cancer.

• Be especially wary of dietary supplements promoted for weight loss, athletic performance, and sexual enhancement. Many of them have been recalled because they were adulterated with prescription drugs used for those indications.

• Be sure to tell your doctor if you take supplements. Many of them interact with prescription and over-the-counter drugs or have side effects that can mimic those of prescribed drugs you're taking. And excessive bleeding can occur during surgical procedures as a result of taking certain supplements.

• Report any side effect you have had, or think you had, directly to the FDA at 800-332-1088. This is the only way to help create a safety net. It is estimated that less than 1 percent of adverse reactions are ever reported.

PREBIOTIC FIBER

Q *I recently saw Fiber Choice fruit-flavored "prebiotic" fiber supplements at a store. Prebiotic? What's that?*

A Probiotic fiber might promote better bowel function by spurring the growth of healthy bacteria in the digestive tract. The supplements you saw contain a type of soluble fiber called inulin, which has prebiotic properties. Inulin supplements may help certain people by improving digestive health and boosting the absorption of certain nutrients. But they may also cause bloating and gas. In general, unless your doctor has suggested a fiber supplement—because you can't eat high-fiber food or have a condition that requires high fiber intake—it's better to get your fiber from food. A diet rich in fruit, vegetables, legumes, and whole grains provides a natural mix of all beneficial fiber types, both soluble and insoluble, helping you maximize benefits.

Water: Diet and safety

TONIC-WATER TEMPERANCE?

Q *My doctor told me to drink tonic water with quinine to help soothe leg cramps. But an issue of* Consumer Reports on Health *from several years back said the drug quinine is no longer FDA-approved for anything except malaria because of safety concerns. Should I be worried about drinking tonic water?*

A Probably not. The worrisome adverse effects—notably fever, nausea, vomiting, diarrhea, auditory and visual hallucinations, and, rarely, potentially fatal allergic reactions—are uncommon and occur only when people consume the equivalent of the typical drug dosage of quinine. Even if you chose one of the tonic-water brands highest in quinine, you'd have to consistently drink almost two liters a day to reach that dosage. And even then, the risk is small. Note that a few people are sensitive to quinine and shouldn't drink tonic water at all; fortunately, since there's no way to tell beforehand, such sensitivity is rare.

WATER AND DIETING

Q *Some diet programs have you drink 10 glasses of water a day. What's the point?*

A The main reason is to prevent kidney stones. Very-low-calorie diet programs can break down the body's protein stores, resulting in excess uric acid in the blood. When excreted in the urine, the excess acid can lead to kidney stones. Drinking large quantities of fluids dilutes the urine and lessens the likelihood of stones. In addition, drinking water frequently can stop hunger contractions of the stomach and create a temporary sensation of fullness.

WELL-WATER SAFETY

Q *We recently moved to the country. Is well water automatically better for my family than city water, or can it be just as dangerous? Also, now that we're not drinking fluoridated water, what should I do to keep my family's teeth healthy?*

A Well water is by no means automatically safer than city water. In fact, for well-run city systems supplied by protected reservoirs, the reverse may be true.

The quality of well water depends on what's in the underground aquifer from which it's drawn. Among potential aquifer pollutants are septic-tank seepage, gasoline from leaking underground tanks, agricultural fertilizers and pesticides, road salt, and industrial wastes. To make certain your well is safe, have the water tested by a reputable laboratory. You can also call EPA's Safe Water Hotline, 800-426-4791, or visit *http://water. epa.gov/scitech/drinkingwater/labcert/index.cfm*. Your state health department might test your water for you or suggest a lab to do so. Also check with your local water authority to determine whether periodic testing is advisable.

Make sure the initial test covers fluoride, which occurs naturally in some well water. Children under 14 need fluoride to strengthen their developing teeth. If your water doesn't have the optimal amount, your dentist or pediatrician can prescribe drops or chewable tablets. Using fluoridated toothpaste and fluoride rinses is sufficient to protect against tooth decay in most teenagers and adults.

Weight control

LATEST "FAT BURNER"

Q *Do unroasted coffee-bean supplements really help you lose weight?*

A It's not clear yet. Limited data have suggested that the extract from unroasted or "green" coffee beans may aid in weight loss for obese or overweight patients, possibly due to its chlorogenic acid, an antioxidant that may play a role in glucose and fat metabolism. But the studies have been small and of limited quality, so it's hard to draw meaningful conclusions from them. Like all supplements, unroasted coffee extract hasn't been evaluated for efficacy or safety by the Food and Drug Administration, nor is there any guarantee of its quality. In recent tests of eight green coffee-bean supplements by the group ConsumerLab.com, four products didn't contain the expected amount of extract, and one had no detectable extract at all.

HOW TO STOP LOSING WEIGHT

Q *I'm a 62-year-old man who has lost 15 pounds in two months through diet and exercise. I feel great, but when I reach my desired weight, how do I adjust my regimen to avoiding losing more pounds? Should I let my appetite decide when to level off? Or should I increase the calories and fat in my diet?*

A First, don't stop exercising: It provides numerous health benefits beyond weight control. As for food, try following your appetite. If you're like most people, your brain will automatically regulate your calorie intake—and thus your weight—by controlling your hunger. However, that self-regulating system doesn't work for everyone, because of differences in metabolism and heredity. If you continue to lose weight, you should see a doctor. If you start gaining weight, you may have to cut back on fat and calories or try to burn more calories by exercising longer or harder.

MIDDLE-AGE SPREAD

Q *What is the best way to control middle-age spread: diet, exercise, or both?*

A Both—including exercises to tone muscles and burn fat. People acquire body fat in two distinct patterns. In so-called middle-age spread, fat accumulates in a "spare tire" around the belly, giving you an apple shape. The other distribution is pear-shaped, with fat deposited around the hips rather than the waist. Men are most often "apples"; women, most often "pears."

Exercises that strengthen your stomach muscles, such as sit-ups, can help restrain a bulging belly. But they won't reduce the amount of abdominal fat. The only way to take that fat off and keep it off is to eat fewer calories and do exercises like biking, jogging, swimming, and walking, which burn a lot of calories.

IS BEING SKINNY RISKY?

Q *I don't smoke or have any disease. But my body mass index is in the underweight range. Is that unhealthy?*

A Almost surely not. Body mass index (BMI) was devised to measure obesity, and conclusions drawn about thinness have been misleading. The BMI is calculated by multiplying weight in pounds by 705, dividing by height in inches, then dividing by height again. A BMI of 30 and over is considered obese, 25 through 29 overweight, and 20 through 24 ideal. Scores below 20 are considered underweight because studies have linked them to increased risk of premature death. But that's almost certainly because disease, eating disorders, or malnourishment make some people thin, not because thinness makes people susceptible to deadly diseases. And while a low BMI may slightly increase your risk of developing osteoporosis, you can counter that by getting enough exercise and calcium. Note that BMI may be misleading in another way: People who have bulky muscles may be classified as overweight even if they have little body fat.

SKINNY PEOPLE, FATTY DIET

Q *Since I'm very thin and want to gain weight, I eat plenty of fatty foods. Will my low weight keep my blood-cholesterol levels down despite the high-fat diet?*

A No. A high-fat diet can increase blood-cholesterol levels in thin people as well as in heavy people. The body's tendency to convert dietary fat into blood cholesterol is entirely separate from its tendency to deposit that fat on your waist or thighs. To try to gain weight, increase your consumption of a variety of foods, not just fatty ones. But remember that thin people can have just as much trouble gaining weight and keeping it on as most heavy people have losing weight and keeping it off.

FLABBY ABDOMEN

Q *How can a person lose fat from the lower abdomen when the rest of the body is relatively lean?*

A There's really no such thing as "spot reduction" exercises that zero in on fat in a specific area. When you work out, you use energy produced by burning fat from all over your body—not just around the muscles doing the most work. So aside from burning a few calories, all that exercises such as sit-ups do is strengthen your abdominal muscles and help hold your gut in.

However, studies do suggest that people losing weight—whether through any sort of exercise, calorie reduction, or both—tend to shed abdominal fat faster than fat from other parts of the body. That's good news, not only for your appearance, but also for your health: Abdominal fat seems to pose a higher risk of coronary heart disease than fat deposited in other areas.

WHY THIN PEOPLE DON'T GAIN

Q *Why do some people stay too thin even though they're trying to gain weight?*

A Like their heavy counterparts, thin people seem to be programmed to remain close to a certain weight. They might be able to add pounds by cultivating patently unhealthy habits—avoiding exercise and gorging on high-calorie foods. But most thin people who tried to live that dieter's dream would actually find it hard to stay underactive and overindulgent. Eventually, they'd revert to their usual habits and usual weight. Thin people do have another option: muscle-building exercises. But again, the extra weight will be lost if they stop pumping iron.

✚ *Office* **Visit**

Explaining unexplained weight loss

TEARS WELLED UP IN MY PATIENT'S EYES AS SHE STEPPED OFF my office scale. "I've lost another two pounds," she sobbed. "It's got to be something serious." An 80-year-old recently widowed former painter, she had always enjoyed good health. That is, until about six months earlier, when she began losing weight without meaning to. In her younger years she had always been a bit stout, with many unsuccessful attempts at dieting, so she was pleased at first with her new look and the improved fit of her clothes. But after losing 12 pounds, she began to worry about dire underlying problems. Her dietary patterns had not changed, she did not appear to be depressed, and she had no symptoms that might have pointed me in one direction or another in my attempt to find a cause. Her situation was not unusual; unintentional weight loss affects about 15 to 20 percent of people over the age of 65.

Is it cancer?

Those of us who have tried to lose weight on purpose know how frustrating and difficult it can be, but unintentional weight loss is even more problematic and prompts fears of dread diseases with fatal outcomes. Those fears have some basis in reality. For many, thoughts turn to cancer, especially malignancies that are occult, meaning they cause no symptoms until they reach an advanced stage. The most common are cancers of the pancreas, lung, ovary, kidney, and lymphatic system. The medical literature is of no help in this regard. In several studies on involuntary weight loss, cancer was present in as little as 6 percent of the patients to as much as 38 percent of them. One mildly encouraging finding was that if a patient did have cancer, it usually showed up during an initial evaluation, which included a careful medical history, a physical examination, laboratory tests, X-rays, gastrointestinal endoscopy, and an abdominal sonogram. To put it another way, if that first battery of tests didn't yield a cancer diagnosis, the involuntary weight loss probably had another cause.

Of those other known causes of involuntary weight loss, nonmalignant diseases, especially those resulting in the malabsorption of nutrients from the intestinal tract, such as adult celiac disease, can elude detection on the initial round of tests. So can occult infections of the heart valves or other sites. An overactive thyroid and diabetes are usually more obvious.

But high on anyone's list of unintentional weight loss causes are psychosocial factors that include bereavement, loneliness, depression, and a loss or major reduction of income, either alone or in combination.

No cause found

Unintentional weight loss remains unexplained in as many as 28 percent of patients, despite extensive investigation, for follow-up periods from six months to three years. Yet it's associated with increased sickness and death within the following year or two. In a classic experiment done in the 1990s, a group of older men deliberately lost weight by means of a calorie-restricted diet. Later, when they were allowed to eat as much as they wanted, they had great difficulty regaining even a portion of the lost weight compared with younger men who had gone through the same low-calorie weight-loss program. Some researchers have termed this phenomenon the "anorexia of aging."

Many older people complain about not being able to eat as much as they did in their youth without feeling overly full. Dental problems, decreases in smell and taste, and delayed stomach emptying can contribute to limited food intake. Liquid vitamin-protein-calorie supplements like *Ensure* are of little help and can be so filling they compete with the intake of real food. So-called appetite stimulants, such as cyproheptadine and megestrol—both prescribed off-label—have not been found to be effective, and the FDA has not approved any drugs specifically to increase appetite in the elderly.

As for my patient, a battery of the usual blood tests plus a few esoteric ones netted us nothing except a small degree of reassurance, which was further bolstered by one or two normal imaging procedures. Consultations with a colleague yielded no further information. With encouragement, reassurance, and enjoyable dinners with friends, she managed to gain back a few pounds, and her weight has been stable for the past eight months. Whatever its cause, her alarming weight loss has taken a holiday, at least for the time being.

Women's health

BLOOD TEST FOR OVARIAN CANCER

 I keep hearing about a blood test for ovarian cancer. Is it reliable?

A Not very. The test checks the blood level of a protein called CA-125, which is usually elevated in women with ovarian cancer. While that can provide an early diagnosis, the benefit is generally outweighed by the high chance of false alarms. That's because several other conditions also elevate CA-125, including pregnancy, endometriosis (the spread of uterine tissue to other pelvic organs), uterine fibroids, and pelvic inflammatory disease. Women at high risk for ovarian cancer because their mother or sister had it might still want to consider the test because their increased susceptibility may override concerns about false-positive results. The test is mainly used in women being treated for ovarian cancer to track the therapy's progress. All other women should stick with periodic pelvic examinations by a doctor.

SEX PILLS

Q *Are there any alternatives to Viagra that are sold over the counter?*

A None that we can safely recommend. Supplements that claim to enhance male sexual performance don't have to meet the same safety and efficacy standards as prescription medications. And many have been found to be contaminated with prescription drugs, including sildenafil, the active ingredient in *Viagra*. Even "natural" sex enhancers can be dangerous; the herb yohimbe, for example, can cause potentially fatal changes in heart rate and blood pressure. Since supplements can interact with prescription drugs, you should always tell your doctor which ones you currently take or plan to take.

ANNUAL PAP SMEAR

Q *How often should a woman get a Pap smear? And what time of month gives the most accurate results?*

A The venerable Pap smear is one of the most important cancer-detection tests, and in our March 2013 Ratings of cancer screening tests, it received our highest rating for women age 21 to 65. A woman should begin having a Pap smear beginning at age 21 every three years through age 30. Women 30 to 65 can go five years if they had HPV (human papillomavirus) testing when they had their Pap smear. Some gynecologists recommend that women at high risk for cervical cancer be tested even more frequently. (Risk factors include multiple sex partners, certain viruses, venereal warts, and smoking.) Pap smears should not be done during the menstrual period. Some recent data suggest that the test is more accurate during the first half of the cycle if you use oral contraceptives. Midcycle is preferred for most other menstruating women. Regardless of the timing, the technician reading the smear must know if you're taking oral contraceptives or estrogen replacement therapy, and the date of your last menstrual period. Women 65 and older who have had at least three normal pap smears in the past 10 years can stop.

SOY AND BREAST CANCER

Q *I have read that the plant estrogens in soybeans may not be safe for postmenopausal women. My oncologist "felt" that consuming soy was "probably" OK. But having had breast cancer, I don't want to follow feelings or "probably."*

A There's not enough hard evidence to make a definitive statement about the health effects of soy-based estrogens. Several observational studies have found that women who consumed the most plant-based estrogens have a lower risk of breast cancer than women who consumed the least. But there's also at least a theoretical concern that those compounds may stimulate tumor growth in women who have estrogen-responsive breast cancer, particularly postmenopausal women.

The overall pattern of your diet matters more than any one particular food. It's probably OK for women—including postmenopausal women with breast cancer—to eat soy-based foods in moderate amounts as part of a balanced diet (low in animal fat, high in produce). However, our consultants feel that those women—as well as women at high risk for breast cancer— should talk with their doctors before consuming large amounts of soy.

BREAST TENDERNESS

Q *For breast tenderness, my gynecologist recommended 1,200 IU of vitamin E a day for life. He also recommended cutting back on caffeine. Are those treatments effective?*

A There's no convincing evidence that eliminating caffeine or adding vitamin E helps relieve breast pain, which is usually caused by fluid retained just before menstruation. If your pain does precede menstruation, you might try taking a mild diuretic during the few days before your period. An over-the-counter pain reliever and a supportive bra might also help.

ANTIBIOTICS AND YEAST

Q *Every time I take antibiotics, I end up with a yeast infection. How can I prevent this?*

A Whether or not yeast infections can be prevented is a matter of controversy. Since you always seem to get an infection when taking antibiotics, you could try using an antifungal vaginal cream at the same time. Those creams include butoconazole (*Mycelex-3*) and clotrimazole (*Gyne-Lotrimin-3*, *Mycelex-7*, and generic), all sold over the counter. And eating yogurt with active cultures may help as well.

CONTRACEPTION ALERT

Q *Is it true that the antibiotic tetracycline* (Achromycin) *can reduce the effectiveness of birth-control pills?*

A Yes. So can a long list of other common drugs (and even an herb). Those include the antibiotics amoxicillin, ampicillin

(*Principen*), doxycycline (*Vibramycin* and generic), penicillin, and rifampin (*Rifadin, Rimactane,* and generic); the anticonvulsant drugs carbamazepine (*Carbatrol, Epitol, Tegretol,* and generic), phenytoin (*Dilantin, Phenytex,* and generic), and primidone (*Mysoline* and generic); the antifungal medication griseofulvin (Grifulvin); and the antidepressant herb St. John's wort. All those agents can boost the production of certain liver enzymes that help the body eliminate estrogens, which are the active ingredients in many birth-control pills. So in theory, they could all reduce protection against pregnancy. In practice, unintentional pregnancies have been reported in women taking certain medications together with the pill. To be safe, use an alternative or additional form of birth control if you're taking any of these agents while using an oral contraceptive.

HOT FLASHES AND DIURETICS

Q *I've heard that the water-ridding properties of diuretics such as* Dyazide *(triamterene/hydrochlorothiazide) make it essential to drink plenty of fluids during hot weather to prevent dehydration. Since the hot flashes that accompany menopause can also make you sweat, would that likewise lead to a dehydration risk from diuretics?*

A No. Menopausal hot flashes are caused by temporarily dilated blood vessels in the skin. While that may make you sweat, you won't lose a significant amount of water, even if you're taking a diuretic.

Index

Allergies, 3–5
    antihistamines, 5
    colloidal silver risks, 205–206
    dermatitis, contact, 183–184
    dust mites, 3
    flowers, less allergenic, 3–4
    food allergies, 4, 65
    hives, 181–182, 184
    shots, 4
    stove risks, 19
Arm, leg, and foot ailments, 5–13
    athlete's foot, 6
    burning sensation in feet, 9
    cold extremities, 7
    corn removal, 7–8
    edema, 11–13
    toenails, ingrown, 176–177
    toenail fungus, 5
    leg swelling, 8–9, 10
    lymphedema, 10
    numbness in limbs, 8
    numbness in toes, 149
Arthritis and joint and muscle
        disorders, 13–19
    arthritis supplements, 16
    bursitis of the hip, 15
    disjointed fingers, 14–15
    gout, 17–19
    heat vs. cold treatment, 14
    muscle cramps, 16, 109, 113,
        213
    rubs, 15
    weather-related pain, 13
Asthma and lung problems,
        19–23

blood clot in lung, 20
breathlessness, 21–23
change of locales, 20
gas stove risks, 19
smoking, frequency of, 23

Back pain, 24–26
    herniated disk, 24
    lumbar decompression, 25–26
    push-ups, 25
    spinal surgery, 24
    traction therapy, 25
    spinal X-ray risks, 26
Bladder and urinary problems,
        27–29
    diuretics, 27
    nighttime bladder fullness, 28
    overactive bladder, 27, 28
    pelvic exercises, 29
Blood pressure, 29–32
    and high temperatures, 32
    and potassium, 30–31, 89
    blood-pressure drugs and
        impotence, 147–148
    fluctuations, 29, 31
    hypertension (high blood
        pressure), 13, 27, 30, 32
    low blood pressure, 32
    raised systolic pressure, 31–32
    when to check, 30
Bone health, 33–38
    calcium absorption, 33–34
    calcium supplements (See
        Vitamins and supplements)
    height loss, 33

low bone density, 36–38
osteoporosis, 26, 33–35, 36–38
171–172, 196–197, 217
oxalate in tea, 33–34
tailbone pain, 35

Cardiovascular disorders, 38–46
angina, 40, 49
angiogram accuracy, 41
aspirin for heart attacks, 39
atrial fibrillation, 39–40, 42–44
catheter ablation procedure, 40
heart attack and diet, 44–46
heart palpitations, 41
rapid heartbeat, 38, 39–40
stroke prevention, 42–44
Cholesterol, 47–52
and coffee, 52
clogged arteries, 47
HDL vs. LDL, 49–50
HDL-raising foods, 48–49
statin drugs
and consumption of
grapefruit, 49
side effects of, 48
stopping usage, 50
testing, 51
triglycerides, 51–52
Colds (See Respiratory
infections)
Colon and rectal complaints,
53–57
anal itching, 55
bloody stool, 56
bowel movements, infrequent,
54
colon cleansers, 56–57
diarrhea, 187, 213

diverticulosis and diet, 54–55
gas and flatulence, 84, 188,
189–191
hemorrhoids, 53
inflammatory bowel disease,
208
irritable bowel syndrome, 185,
188, 190, 192
soy products, effects of, 84,
187–188
Constipation (See Stomach
ailments)
Cysts, lumps, and tumors, 57–58
acoustic nerve tumors, 98
benign changes in breast, 58
breast tumors and plant
estrogens, 223
dermatofibroma lumps, 57
lipomas, 57–58
lower back tumors, 27, 35
pituitary tumors, 93

Dental care, 59–64
bad breath, 59
calcium supplements (See
Vitamins and supplements)
gum care, 60–61
toothbrush hygiene, 61–62
toothpaste for sensitive teeth,
61
X-rays, 60, 62–64
Diabetes, 65–68
after-dinner drowsiness, 65
aspirin for lowering blood
sugar, 65
diabetes insipidus, 67–68
diabetes mellitus, 66–67
Diet and nutrition, 68–90

balanced meals, 83
bananas, benefits, 71–72
bananas, radiation risk, 89–90
blood-thinning supplements, 43
broccoli, best parts, 82
cheese, hard vs. soft, 81
chicken, sodium in, 68
cholesterol, 47–52, 77, 80–81, 86, 187, 196, 208, 217
cooking vegetables, 77
diet and exercise, 108
dietary supplements, 210–212 (*See Vitamins and supplements*)
eggplant, 72–73
eggs, salmonella risks, 76–77
fats, 51–52, 69
fats for frying, 69
feverfew, 121–122
fiber, digesting, 74
    foods high in, 48, 55
    prebiotic fiber, 212
    types of fiber, 74–75
fruit
    dried fruits, 83
    fruit juice pulp, 72
    sugar in, 87–88
leafy greens and blood-clot risk, 73, 84–85
liquid nutritional supplements, 85
microwave cooking, 79
midnight snacks, 88
mushroom risks, 75
omega-3s
    depletion in smoked foods, 70
    sources, 86

onions, benefits, 80–81
peeling fruits and vegetables, 71
pesticides on fruits and vegetables, 71
potatoes, baked vs. sweet, 73–74
produce, nutrient degradation in, 76
protein, from plants, 78
resveratrol, in red wine and grapes, 88–89
root vegetable tops (leaves), 80
salt substitutes, 89
smoked meat risks, 78–79
soy nuts, 85–86
soy products and gas, 84, 187
vegetable and fruit consumption, 77–78
water, bottled vs. tap, 69–70
water diets, 213–214
water, when to drink, 87
yams vs. sweet potatoes, 81–82
Doctors, 90–97
    describing your symptoms, 91–93
    doctors' fees, haggling over, 93–95
    doctors of osteopathy vs. doctors of medicine, 90
    waiting room hints and tips, 95–97
Drugs (*See Medications*)

Ear problems, 98–99
    and air travel, 98–99
    cotton swabs, 99
    tinnitus, causes, 98
Exercise and fitness, 108–116

aerobic cramping, 113–114
aerobic exercise, 108, 113
ankle weight risks, 108–109
Body Mass Index (BMI), 111
cardiovascular fitness, 112
exercise and constipation, 185
exercise and metabolism rate, 109
exercise for weight loss, 108, 112–113
muscles, electrical stimulation of, 110
resting heart rate, 115, 116
resistance exercise, 114
rowing machines, 115
strength training for older people, 114
sweating, benefits of, 109–110
swimming, 114–115
weight lifting, proper breathing during, 116
workout timing, 110–111
Eye care, 100–107
cholesterol deposits on eyelid, 102
computer use and vision, 102–103
contact lens infections, 104–105
contact lens rinsing, 104
dry-eye syndrome, 105–107
flashbulb risks, 101
floaters, 100–101
nonprescription reading glasses, 103–104
sunglasses (plastic), 100
twitching eyelid, 103
vision supplements, 101–102

Fiber *(See Diet and nutrition)*
Flatulence *(See Colon and rectal problems)*

Gout, 17–19
diagnosis and treatment, 18–19
gout and diet, 17–18
gout and mushrooms, 75
quick onset of, 46

Hair care, 117–119
dandruff shampoo, 117–118
ear, nose, and eyebrow hair, 119
electrolysis, 118
hair loss and vitamin A, 118–119
hair loss, women's 117
Headaches, 120–124
carbon monoxide poisoning, as symptom of, 91
concussion, as symptom of, 156-159
Cushing's disease, as symptom of, 93
during sexual activity, 121
from blow to the head, 150
hangover prevention, 120–121
ice-cream headache, 120
Lyme disease, as symptom of, 129
migraines and feverfew, 121–122
migraine triggers, 122–124
Health fears and risks, 125–131
Alzheimer's disease, 131
body temperature, 128
fiberglass, 128
germ contact, 127

giving blood, risks and
    benefits, 125
low blood sugar, 127–128
Lyme disease, 129–131
night sweats, 125
smoking-cessation risks,
    126–127
tetanus, 126
Heartburn, 132–133
    heartburn medications, length
        of use, 132
    heartburn medications and
        nutrient loss, 133
    surgery for heartburn, 132–133

Liver disorders, 134
    Gilbert's syndrome, 134
    liver-damaging drugs, 5, 141–
        142
    liver-disease testing, 134
    mushrooms and liver cancer, 75

Medical procedures, 135–140
    angiography, noninvasive,
        136–137
    biopsy pain, 136
    difficult blood draws, 135
    health center screenings, 137
    stress tests, 135–136, 138–140
Medications, 140–143
    adult immunizations, 198
    allergy shots, 4
    antibiotic salves, 142–143
    antihistamines, 5
    aspirin, no-name, 142
    blood-thinning supplements,
        143
    expiration dates, 140–141

liver-damaging drugs, 141–142
low bone-density drugs, 36–38
Reye's syndrome, aspirin risks,
    140
Men's health, 144–148
    enlarged prostate, 145–146
    impotence and blood-pressure
        drugs, 147–148
    Peyronie's disease, 148
    prostate health and sexual
        activity, 147
    prostate screening, 144–145
    prostatectomy and infertility,
        144
    pumpkin seeds for prostate
        relief, 146
    vasectomy and prostate cancer,
        145

Neurological problems, 149–159
    essential tremor, 149, 151–153
        treatment, 149, 153
    head injury and concussion,
        150–151, 156–159
    neuropathies, 154–156
    sciatica, 149, 155
    slapping gait, 150
Nose, mouth, and throat
    disorders, 159–170
    burning mouth, 159
    dry mouth, chronic, 162–163
    nosebleeds, 164–165
    postnasal drip, 167
    rhinitis, vasomotor, 164
    salivary gland disorders, 163
    Schatzki's ring, 170
    smell, loss of, 166
    sore-throat treatments, 160, 162

swallowing difficulties,
167–168, 168–170
taste, loss of, 166–167
thrush, 165
tongue disorders, 163–164
Parenting and pregnancy, 171–
173
breast-feeding, osteoporosis
risks, 171–172
postpartum depression, 172–
173
post-pill pregnancies, 172
safety belts while pregnant,
171
Prostate problems *(See Men's
health)*

Respiratory infections, 173–174
bronchial infections and
smoking, 173
colds, treating with antibiotics,
173–174

Skin care, 174–184
acne, adult, 176
bags under the eyes, 178
blackhead removal, 180–181
cucumbers and skin, 180
facial exercises to reduce
wrinkles, 177–178
flushed face, 179–180
hives, 181–182, 184
hydrogen peroxide for cuts,
175
itching, 178, 181, 182–184
manicures, and infections,
174–175
nail fungus and infections, 5–6,

174–175
rosacea, laser treatment, 179
skin spots (vitiligo), treatment,
177
sunscreen, expiration, 175
toenails, ingrown, 176–177
Stomach ailments, 185–193
artificial sweeteners and
stomach pain, 186
constipation, 191–193
and exercise, 185
flatulence, 46, 187, 188,
189–191
gastritis pain, 185–186
irritable bowel syndrome, 185,
188, 190, 192
soy milk and heartburn relief,
187–188
testing for bacterial infections,
186–187
ulcer-causing bacteria, 186–
187

Thyroid problems, 194–197
goiters and diet, 197
thyroid disease, 195–197
thyroid-drug dependency, 194
underactive thyroid, 194

Vaccines, 198–204
adult immunizations, 198
flu vaccine, 198–199
pertussis shot, advisability of,
200
pertussis vaccine and
Medicare, 199
pneumonia vaccine, 200
shingles and stroke, 201

shingles vaccine, 201
vaccinations, importance of, 202–204
Vitamins and supplements, 204–212
  B-complex vitamins, 47, 75, 77, 78, 83, 204
  calcium, 33, 34, 35, 59–60, 73, 78, 80, 81, 172, 188, 192, 217
  colloidal silver risks, 205–206
  dietary supplements, dangers, 210–212
  folate (folic acid), 79, 80, 207
  iron, 78, 192, 204
  lycopene, 73
  mad-cow disease, risk, 205
  magnesium, 82, 133
  potassium, 30–31, 72, 80, 82, 85, 89, 90, 169
  protein, 73, 75, 78, 81, 82, 85–86, 187
  vitamin A , 73, 77, 80, 83, 118–119, 204, 208
    B6, 72, 90
    B12, 47, 133, 154, 206–208
    C, 18, 72, 73, 77, 80, 82, 83, 204
    D, 33, 188, 208, 209
    E, 83, 85, 204, 224
    K, 73, 80, 84, 208
  vitamins and the flu, 204
  vitamins, fat-soluble, 208–209
    water-soluble, 83
  zinc, 204

Water, 213–214
  bottled vs. tap, 69–70

  intake while dieting, 213–214
  tonic-water safety, 213
  well-water safety, 214
  when to drink, 87
Weight control, 215–221
  abdominal fat, 217–218
  Body Mass Index (BMI), 111, 216–217
  coffee-bean supplements, 215
  exercise and weight loss, 108, 215–216
  weight and cholesterol, 217
  weight gain in middle age, 216
  weight loss, unintentional, 216–217, 218, 219–221
Women's health, 221–225
  birth-control pills and antibiotics, 224–225
  breast cancer and soy products, 223
  breast tenderness and vitamin E, 224
  hot flashes and diuretics, 225
  ovarian cancer blood test, 221–222
  Pap smear, annual, 222
  sex supplements, 222
  yeast infections and antibiotics, 224